"This work serves as a gift to o
journey and awakening to thi
as a down to earth focus and direction, ....
daily lifework world of nursing and nurses."

**Jean Watson,** PhD, RN, AHN-BC, FAAN, LL (AAN)
Founder/Director Watson Caring Science Institute, Boulder, Colorado
Distinguished Professor/Dean Emerita
University of Colorado Denver, College of Nursing

"An urgently needed call to nurse leaders and a roadmap for all
nurses to find, be, and engage from authentic caring self. Both
inspiring and resourceful, this text demonstrates how to transform
self and expand organizational influence for changing the hearts,
minds and skills of the healthcare workforce."

**Sara Horton-Deutsch,** PhD, RN, FAAN, ANEF, Caritas Coach
Professor
University of San Francisco School of Nursing and Health Professions
Adjunct Professor at University of Colorado, College of Nursing

"Through years of hard work, introspection, and dedication to the
most trusted of the healing professions, Pat McClendon reminds us
all that caring is the heart and soul of nursing leadership."

**JoAnne Auger,** RN, CHPPN, Caritas Coach

"For those who are less familiar with caring science and its place in
today's healthcare, this book provides an honest description of how
one nurse leader traveled beyond organizational culture trends to
engage nurses in creating meaning in daily work. Pat's approach to
engaging nurses moves beyond superficial scripting and promotes
satisfying dialogue between leaders and bedside nurses. More
importantly, she identifies ways for nurse leaders to infuse routine
activities with caring practices so nurses thrive in the challenging
healthcare environment."

**Caroline Etland,** PhD, RN, CNS, AOCN, ACHPN
Associate Professor, University of San Diego

"I have been in nursing leadership for quite a while, and I couldn't put this memoir down. It was just what I needed - inspiring and helpful."

**Cindy Damboise,** MSN, MHA, RN, CCRN, PCCN
Clinical Manager Medical/Surgical/Orthopedics
Community hospital in Southern California

"This book is timely as the World Health Organization (WHO) has declared 2020 the Year of the Nurse. Nurses have impacted healthcare delivery since Florence Nightingale, yet today's healthcare environments are not always caring. Pat provides new ways to authenticity, self-care and caring interactions with patients and each other. She reminds us why we became nurses, and how to share our voices and our stories. Pat McClendon's beautiful and authentic story is one we can learn from. A must read for every nurse leader!"

**Michelle Goldbach,** DNP, MHA, RN, CHPN
Clinical Manager Palliative Care and Pediatric Hospice Programs
San Diego, California

"I have had the privilege of being inspired by a few mentors in my career. Fierce nurses who have shown me how to embrace vulnerability and passion for patient care and self-care. Pat McClendon continues to stand out. This book illustrates that who we are is how we lead, how we care, how we show up every day to take care of people who need a nurse in their most vulnerable time. Thank you, Pat, for supporting and honoring this, the greatest of professions."

**Jae Sanders,** MSN, FNP-C, CCD
Orthopedic Practice, Colorado Springs, Colorado

# GETTING REAL ABOUT CARING

## WHAT I DISCOVERED ABOUT AUTHENTIC CARING AS A NURSE LEADER AND ONE STEP FORWARD

PAT MCCLENDON

authorHOUSE

*AuthorHouse™*
*1663 Liberty Drive*
*Bloomington, IN 47403*
*www.authorhouse.com*
*Phone: 1 (800) 839-8640*

*Published by AuthorHouse  03/15/2019*

*ISBN: 978-1-7283-0384-0 (sc)*
*ISBN: 978-1-7283-0383-3 (e)*

*Library of Congress Control Number: 2019902932*

*Print information available on the last page.*

# Contents

To nurse leaders,

The orchestra leaders of health care who influence clinical practice, clinical environments, the patient experience, quality, operations and finance, and most of all, nurses.

# ACKNOWLEDGMENTS

To Jean Watson, for ushering the way.
To Karen Faulis, for showing authenticity and ease in leadership.
To Terry McGoldrick, for being a truth teller.
To David and our daughters, for accompanying me on this journey.

# Preface

As a nurse leader, I failed to lead caring in health care. I've cared for patients, I've studied caring theories and science, and for nearly thirty years, I told myself that I was leading caring. Thinking about caring as a nurse leader has been a constant, prompting me to write about it at different stages in my career. I felt I was selling my soul to the health care industry. I tried to warn other nurses. As a new nurse, I submitted a manuscript to the *American Journal of Nursing*, urging nurses to remain true to themselves and to resist being swallowed up by medicine and health care. I knew even then that I was in trouble. And here I am many years later, unraveling the results.

What I know is that nursing is ever evolving. Nursing's history has paralleled the evolution of the human experience and society's health, healing and caring needs within the consciousness of the time. Currently, society's health, healing, and caring needs reflect wellness consciousness— where authenticity and human connectedness create well-being. Patients are not only seeking medical care in their health care encounters; they are also yearning for authentic connections. And it is nurses to whom they are turning for that connection. We are seeing this play out in patient experience metrics. And yet, nursing leaders, distracted by science, technology, and budgets, are not seeing the alignment between the public's expanding caring expectations and nurses' authentic caring. Jean Watson once wrote of nursing, "The change will come when nursing and nurses are directly aligned with the people they serve" (1999, 46).[1] That alignment is before us, but not enough nursing leaders are rising to it.

Beyond being distracted, there is another reason so many nurse leaders are not rising to the growing demand for authentic caring connection. They don't know how. How do nurse leaders engage in this alignment in the health care industry? The generation of authentic caring is nurse-centric. Authentic caring originates within the nurse, sparks from a connection between the nurse and patient, is cultivated through a nurse's internal resources, and can only be sustained by the nurse. How this exchange happens is personal. We know that stress undermines access to and cultivation of nurses' authenticity. We know that how nurses relate to themselves impacts their authenticity and how they care. We know that nurse engagement requires organizational resources to mitigate the job stressors and nurses' inner resources to navigate personal stressors. And we know that cultivation of nurses' inner resources comes through self-care and reflection. Here is the problem: self-care cannot be mandated or managed by nurse leaders or organizations. This makes it complicated for nurse leaders and organizations to take it on; and yet, we must. Nurses' self-care and caring consciousness not only impact nurses' caring; it also drives their ability to thrive in nursing.

Retention is our twenty-first-century challenge. If attrition trends are not reversed, none of the other worthy priorities nurse leaders are consumed in will matter. Up to 50 percent of new nurses are considering a way out of nursing (Kabcenell, Perlo, and Sakallaris 2016; MacKusick and Minick 2010).[2,3] But we can ebb this tide. Nurses are motivated by their intrinsic desires to help others and rarely by organizations' missions. Nurses find science and technology interesting and challenging, but it's the human connections and caring that bring the sense of purpose and meaning to nurses. The health care industry is a beast to work in and is driving nurse attrition. Caring science is there to usher in better ways that help nurses thrive in nursing. Caring science research has defined caring relationships and has shown that authentic caring has a reciprocal nature. It is life-giving and life-receiving for both the patient and the nurse.

I believe that nurse leaders are nurses' only hope for expanded authentic caring in the health care industry given their common ground. Yet the scary reality is that they are in greater jeopardy than clinical nurses. It's reported that up to 72 percent of nurse leaders were devising their exit plans within a five-year window (Warshawsky and Havens 2014).[4] The nurse leader role is one of the most complex leadership roles across all industries. Nurse leaders are wedged between two major forces—medicine and business—making it difficult to preserve one's sense of nursing identity and integrity. This is the reality for the 410,000 nurse leaders whose nurse followers are 3.1 million strong in the United States. The nurse leader job is full of high-risk, competing demands, fear of failing, and successes that are never enough.

This was my experience as a nurse leader. Like the boiling frog parable, I didn't jump out of the boiling water. Despite having studied caring theory and science at the University of Colorado under Jean Watson in my nursing doctorate education, I did not see caring science as a realistic option as a leader for too long. But then I did.

It was my personal journey into wellness consciousness that saved me—fueled by self-care. I learned that how I live and work, what I focus on, and what I talk about impacts me and those around me. Up until then, I had allowed my leader self to dominate my authentic, caring self. I had to grapple with self-awareness, self-protection, and more before I could find my full authentic voice and lead caring. Until then, I remained stuck within the health care industry, the medicalization of care, and the business demands. How nurse leaders find their authentic leader selves takes many paths, yet there are few stories told. Unraveling where I went wrong and right in my career has catapulted me into telling my story.

Nursing is a complex profession based on our social covenant with society. Nursing leadership's unique challenge is to embolden this covenant. Nursing is the science of designing and providing caregiving individually and collectively. Medicine is the science and business of saving and improving lives. Health care is the business of providing medical services in caring organizations. Nurses juggle it all—saving lives, improving lives, and providing care within health care organizations. Nurses' intrinsic, authentic caring attends to patients' deep human needs, especially in vulnerable life moments. This is not what the health care industry supports and not what nursing leadership resembles. We are not leading authentic caring. We are not role modeling how to thrive in nursing. This is a time for nurse leaders to rise up and lead caring for the well-being of patients, nurses, and society.

Disclaimer: All references to patients are intended to be inclusive of families and individuals who are significant to a patient.

# Introduction

My story is a conversation about my life and career as a nurse, nurse leader, daughter, wife, and mother across four states in stand-alone hospitals, nonprofit and for-profit corporate systems, and through my doctoral nursing education. In this story, I focus on each step in my career, what my world looked like to me, and what held me back from connecting with my purpose. Realizing that who we are is how we lead put me on the path of renewed, authentic connection and caring as a leader.

The purpose of this book is to highlight how the contextual forces within the health care industry impact nurse leaders as told in my story, to urge nurse leaders to give voice to authentic caring in the industry, to draw connections between authentic caring, thriving in nursing and attrition, and to offer one step nurse leaders can use to lead authentic caring. The urgent need for authentic connection and caring in health care calls nurse leaders to see their roles anew. Authentic caring certainly exists today but not at the frequency or systemic level it could if it was seen as a realistic and active part of our work environments. The pace and complexity in nurses' jobs leave many nurses feeling disconnected from their original purpose in being a nurse. Nurse leaders giving voice to authentic caring—with their unique influence and credibility in nurses' work environments—can capture nurses' attention and serve a role in reconnecting nurses to their purpose. Nurse leaders are in the best position to make authentic caring's invisibility visible, and the unrealistic realistic for nurses. The step forward involves episodic and momentary caring engagement conversations—in between patients and meetings—that tap into nurses' existing caring practices. Nurse leaders can help nurses translate their caring experiences into caring literacy and language in real time. These reflective conversations between nurses and leaders introduce a new narrative of mutual authenticity and caring consciousness. This is a real and doable way nurse leaders can ebb the tide of attrition and create a twenty-first-century legacy of nurses thriving in nursing.

# PART I

# GROWING MY NURSE SELF

# CHAPTER 1

# Discovery Begins

Have you ever said something in your career that didn't make sense in the moment, but it had just enough truth that it couldn't be taken back?

It happened to me in a conference room as my fellow leaders and I were taking our seats for a meeting. Several of them were discussing a conflict that had just occurred between two individuals with whom we all worked. The focus of my colleagues' conversation was the importance of being respectful and how these people in the conflict had not been respectful. As I listened to them describe the yelling and the personal affronts, I thought that the conflict sounded like an honest exchange. Yes, it was contentious and should have been done in private, but it sounded honest, and that felt positive to me.

So I blurted out, almost absentmindedly, "Respect is highly overrated."

My colleagues' eyes all turned to me. Their faces seemed horrified by my statement. I felt the air go out of the room. I was stunned that I had said it, mainly because I knew that what

I said had violated our team's unspoken norms. At the same time, I felt there was some truth in what I had said, so I didn't try to backtrack or explain myself. I continued in the swirl of my inner thoughts. Self-judgment took hold, and I shut down. We went on with the meeting as if nothing had happened.

My dismissive statement about respect and my relationship with my peers bothered me for some time. It disrupted my truth-teller self-image. I had always been proud of myself for speaking truth. There was no straight talk or open communication that day, or in the days that followed. I never did explain my thoughts behind my statement. My inner dialogue revolved around, *Of course I know the importance of respect. Why did I feel so threatened and exposed? Why can't I resolve this with my team?* Over time this confusion put me on the road of self-discovery. It started with me seeing the impact of my patterns of avoidance and self-protection in my relationships and in others around me. Knowing how to have crucial conversations with my coworkers escaped me for several more years. I wasn't ready for that until I strengthened my inner resources through self-care. That came with time.

Conflict avoidance and self-protection hold us back from what matters most. They stifle cultivation of our inner resources that help us grow, heal, and connect with others. Our inner resources involve self-awareness, self-acceptance, nonjudgment, gratitude, vulnerability, joy, and more—all the things that lead to authentic connections and thriving in nursing. Learning to cultivate my inner resources and then navigate relationships more openly and honestly amid threats and tensions got me to a place of willingness to see and be in the world differently.

# CHAPTER 2

# My Nurse Origins

My path to nursing was a pragmatic one. After completing a degree in anthropology, I pursued nursing for job and life security based my mother's nursing career. My mom never intended to have a nursing career. She became a registered nurse (RN) because it was required in the 1930s in order to be an airline flight attendant. The airlines had RNs as attendants then to allay the public's fear of flying. After her three years of nurses' training, my mother flew for one year before getting married. Twenty years later, because of life circumstances, she needed a job. She returned to nursing for financial security for our family. To a little girl, that made a deep impression.

## My Nursing School

Student life at the University of Oklahoma (OU) and across the country in the mid-1970s was about a growing social consciousness spurred by political protests over the draft, civil rights, and sexism. My thirst to understand the world and events started in high school and drew me to major in anthropology. My degree in anthropology contributed to my worldview, which set the stage for my nursing education. The nursing faculty at OU was also of the times; they were almost militant in their definition and defense of nursing. They emphasized nursing theories and theorists and the importance of growing nursing science. Their unified mission made clear that nursing was a separate and distinct discipline from medicine. This foundation of nursing's autonomy fit right into my social consciousness and nursing identity then and now. Nursing's struggle within the medical and patriarchal dominance in the health care industry continues today.

This is why Jean Watson surprised me in 2002, when I was sitting on the floor at her side at Naropa University in Boulder, Colorado, in a Caring in Action seminar where she included medicine when referencing caring practices. Her point was that human caring is foundational to all health care disciplines and humanity. I knew then that my understanding of caring was being expanded.

## Mom's Nursing Career

Mom had always been a wise, strong woman whom I idolized through my childhood. My dad was an alcoholic. Their marriage started out full of promise when he graduated from dental school, but life provided challenges. When the marriage hit bottom, a neighbor (an RN) suggested that Mom enter an RN refresher course at the local hospital. This changed her life. It's amazing that these courses can fill the knowledge gap in such short time periods. Life experiences were on my mom's side; after a few years of working, she was asked to participate in the development of the new critical-care programs and units in her hospital.

While my mom was finding her way in the workforce, my dad's cardiovascular health was deteriorating, associated with high blood pressure, heavy alcohol by night, and amphetamines (self-prescribed) by day. At age forty-nine, Daddy had a stroke in his dental office. Knowing his drug and alcohol routine, his doctors were resistant to admit him to the hospital; they were convinced that he just needed to "dry out." And so Daddy was brought home by ambulance from the emergency room, unable to walk, talk, eat, or drink independently; he was awake, alert, and devastated. I was thirteen years old as I stood watching my dad struggle to talk, then try to use his hands to communicate with me, unable to coordinate either. All the while I was listening to my mom on the phone in the other room negotiating a plan to get him back into the hospital for diagnosis and treatment. She had to argue his case with the physicians, Daddy's affluent aunts—who had raised him since his parents' deaths when he was thirteen—and with the insurance companies, whose premium payments had lapsed under Daddy's management. Boy, did I see patriarchy in action; it was my mom against the world, and she prevailed. After he was admitted, it was confirmed that he had had a stroke, and his insurance covered the stay. This was in December of 1963, just a couple of weeks after Kennedy's assassination. My worldview was taking shape.

Daddy died three weeks later after another cluster of strokes. By this time, Mom had gotten him moved to a Veteran's Administration hospital, where he was scheduled for rehabilitation and the costs would continue to be covered. My mom and brother were with him—watching a football game on television on New Year's Day—when he died. During these weeks, my mom snuck me in to see Daddy in both hospitals cloaked in a big raincoat. Visitor rules did not allow children at any time. I learned that health care, even then, was complicated, and I felt that every family needed a nurse to help them navigate it. Nurses were the honorable ones in my view; I was predestined for nursing.

When I was in high school, Mom became the head nurse of the critical care unit she had helped develop. Several years later, when I was in college, she was asked to step down from that position. The nurses who had thrived under her tough love leadership during those early years were demanding more respect from the physicians and more money from the organization. Mom's nursing was not an independent discipline and profession. There was no theory or science. Hers was a practical service that supported medicine and hospitals. I think Mom saw the nurses' demands as a personal affront; she was hurt. In Mom's eyes, she had mentored each of these nurses through their coming of age as critical care nurses and through their personal life dramas. But at that point, she couldn't hear what the nurses were saying. Listening to her stories, I knew she wanted me to understand her point, that the organization had given them great opportunities and they should be more grateful. As a college student in the '70s, I sympathized with what the nurses were saying, so I avoided taking sides. I just listened. That frustrated her.

After her demotion in critical care, Mom worked clinically in the post-anesthesia care unit for the last eight years of her career. As her hospital expanded, the nursing administrators there needed to figure out how to integrate new graduates straight into their critical care units, and they needed a new grad to be their test case. The nursing administrators—still close friends of my mom—all knew I was graduating and asked her if I would be willing to be their test case. As a proud mom, she was thrilled, and I was too. What an opportunity. In that four-month test program, I gained a rapid knowledge download in a clinically progressive organization, along with skill development and one-on-one support in exchange for my feedback on their residency program design.

I witnessed these critical care nurses' independence in managing patients' activities of daily living. They challenged the physicians in progressing patients' activity levels despite the big, bulky equipment and tubes of the times. We problem solved how to get patients out of bed, to urinate on their own, and to drink and eat as soon as possible, while the physicians focused on the rapidly changing medical aspects of care. The physicians followed the nurses' knowledge and ingenuity regarding bowel, bladder, and activity levels around the medical care advancements. It was a wonderful clinical setting to launch my practice. I thank Mom for this.

Later when I was in nurse leadership positions, Mom would ask me about my day, eager to hear all about it. My stories were typical ones, professional identity and autonomy, demands by physicians, and appropriate pay for nurses. She loved nothing more than to listen to me, but my stories seemed to trigger her into reminiscing how the nurses had wronged her when she was demoted from her head-nurse position. She never got over this, and maybe she never forgave me for not supporting her more. I quickly learned that I had to be careful about what work stories I chose to talk about with her. Sometimes her hurt would surface in a sarcastic joke toward me: "If you're so smart, why haven't you figured this out?" Well, the fact was, I knew I needed help in figuring out a lot of things as the years progressed, as a wife, a mother, and a nurse leader.

# CHAPTER 3

# My Clinical Years

In the late '70s my husband, David, and I traveled back and forth across the country for his graduate education. We went from Oklahoma to Ohio University for his director training in theatre, and then three years later, we moved on to California for his professional internship. In the time span of six years, I worked clinically in three states in medical surgical and critical care units. It always surprised me how different and the same nursing practice was across the country.

## Out of Oklahoma and into Ohio

For David and I, leaving Oklahoma was one goal that drew us together, knowing that there was more to experience beyond our home state. Ohio University is in Athens, Ohio. It is set in the Appalachian Mountains that are beautiful. There, he and I experienced two distinct worlds—him thriving in academia, and me working in a small rural hospital in Appalachia. I had to shift from critical care to medical surgical care immediately. Thankfully my organizational skills from working as a nurse aide in long-term care and on a surgical cancer unit while in college served me well. I was able to survive the large patient assignments. And I enjoyed working with the staff who had roots in the Ohio Valley region. My first charge nurse position was there on the evening shift on the surgical unit. What a great shift—the daytime to myself, and social and sleep time after work. On this shift, nurses built relationships. Of course, the average length of stay was probably eight days, and the patients were only really sick for two or three of those days! The rest of the time was for building their strength and storytelling. Listening to these people's life stories was a delight.

I gravitated to two docs who were mentors and muses to me. Both were wise and kind and loved to teach as they rounded. Dr. Gawande was a urologist, and the other was a general surgeon. They each had hobbies they talked about. One played tennis often, and the other updated me on the sewing he did, once he found out that I sewed. Being a small university town, they knew their patients' lives and families and often shared key information that gave dimension to the patients' plans of care.

Many of the patients' stories are still with me. I will always remember the grief and helplessness of an elderly woman, admitted for malaise and failure to thrive, and her husband (a college professor) who didn't know how to help her. She was a proper, white-haired woman who wore pearls. She talked at length about her inability to console her grown son whose son had just been killed in New York City. A fire escape had spontaneously released down upon him while he was walking home from high school. I was able to listen to her off and on through my shift. Now being a parent of grown children, I remember her story whenever I feel helpless. There were moments of triumph, like when a family used my map of the hospital and a planned, narrow timetable to sneak their dog in to be with his beloved owner as she was dying. That dog snuggled right into her arms until the end. That brought healing to all of us. And there were heartbreaking cases, characteristic of a simpler way of life. One young guy refused to seek treatment after his laparotomy that revealed cancer throughout. He could not imagine traveling "all the way up" to Columbus (seventy-four miles) for further diagnosis and treatment at Ohio State. We had to surrender to his choice. And there was the little elderly lady covered in black soot each time she was admitted during the winter months to have her bowels evacuated because it was too difficult for her to get to the outhouse in the hills in the severe cold. She brought funny stories with each admission. And then there was the saddest case of all, watching over a two-month span the progressive march of amyotrophic lateral sclerosis (ALS) up a woman's body as she lay smiling at her family during evening visits. I remember helping her tell them between breaths about her realization that on one of those days the ALS was going to stop her chest from rising. She died when they were not present. These are the stories that helped me know that I was a part of something bigger than myself. I believe that it was easier to recognize and fully experience these bigger-than-life moments then than it is today at our whirlwind clinical pace.

Even at that slow pace, errors happened. One error was mine in judgment. One of my patients, a strong construction worker in the prime of his life, had returned from the surgery post-nephrectomy in excruciating pain when we transferred him into his bed. I got him settled. He remained stable, so I let him sleep through one turning cycle. When I turned him at the next scheduled time, he was lying in a pool of blood. I almost passed out. He responded, but his vital signs where dropping. Another RN and I stabilized him following Dr. Gawande's clear orders. The patient did well. Dr Gawande's calm response helped me recover my confidence and ability to learn fully from the event.

These memories were given new life thirty-five years later when I happened upon a Public Broadcasting System documentary, *Being Mortal,* one evening in early 2015. I was unpacking boxes after our move to a new house. What made me sit down to watch was the author and narrator, Atul Gawande, referring to Athens, Ohio. "My father was a surgeon in Athens, Ohio," he said. I was stunned. Atul Gawande was Dr. Gawande's son? I had received his book, *Being Mortal,* for Christmas from a friend who knew that I loved *The Checklist Manifesto* by the same Atul Gawande, but the book was still boxed up. I did not know of this father-son connection. I remembered Dr. Gawande talking about his son and daughter when I was in Ohio. And here I was seeing his son talking about how his father had guided him through his end-of-life decision-making—the same Dr. Gawande who had guided me as a young nurse.

## Becoming Adults in San Diego

After David finished his graduate coursework in 1979, we were off to San Diego for his directing internship in professional theatre. We had a choice—New York City or San Diego.

After living through the worst winters the Ohio Valley had on record, I said, "We're going west. I hear it's warm and beautiful there."

And indeed it was. Traveling across the country, through winter storms and the desert, was like a *Grapes of Wrath* scene. We arrived in San Diego in our caravan of David driving a moving truck and me driving our car with our dog and cat, packed to the gills. Seeing San Diego that first time felt like a tropical heaven.

Once we got settled, I started working. My plan for San Diego was to play it safe by not putting myself forward as a critical care nurse since it had been three years since I had worked in a real intensive care unit. As an agency nurse, I got a sense of San Diego's rapid health care growth challenges on my first day. When I walked into the nursing office of a community hospital to sign in and get my medical surgical unit assignment, the staffing clerk and house supervisor both wildly looked up at me and smiled politely. With papers and schedules askew, each had phones to both ears, dialing and talking to nurses and agencies. They were on a mission to find a critical care nurse.

And then, the house supervisor called out to me laughingly, "Have you ever seen the inside of a critical care unit?" I gave a rundown of my clinical experience. We bonded instantly. That was the beginning of my thirteen-year relationship with that community hospital.

San Diego was over-bedded in the '70s and '80s. There were more than twenty hospitals throughout the county with a population of less than two million. This was the result of uncontrolled business investments in health care at the time associated with the anticipated population growth trajectory for San Diego County. My Thomas Map—a book of paper maps by region, the ancestral electronic map—was marked with all the hospital locations. This prepared me for any agency nurse assignment anywhere in the county. The surplus of hospitals attracted a surplus of young, talented physicians of all subspecialties staking their territory in this Shangri-La location. The critical cares felt like freehanded cowboy-medicine arenas, each doc vying to demonstrate their command of the latest science and technology. The wildly fluctuating censuses made staffing a daily roller coaster ride for each hospital and led to in-house staff instability at many. So I stuck with agency nursing for a year, where I could customize my schedule. Agency nursing allowed me to learn the nuances of San Diego's different communities and hospitals, and forced me to grow adaptation skills. I kept coming back to that first community hospital. Once their census stabilized, I hired on as a critical care nurse.

Graduate school was part of my plan, but I had no idea how this was going to happen financially. Our dreams were in motion. We were in one of the most beautiful places in the world, and David was directing Shakespeare in Balboa Park with artists from all over. What more could one ask for? But the routines of adult life were setting in, and I wanted more. It was time to move myself forward. I started researching my school options. My motto became: when in doubt, go back to school.

And indeed I did. This was 1980, and there were only a few masters in science of nursing (MSN) programs in California, and one was at the University of San Diego (USD), a private school that was expensive. A fellow critical care nurse who was in the program encouraged me to go talk to them. As I drove up the road to the campus with white buildings and gilded towers on a hill overlooking San Diego, I thought, *What am I doing here?* My appointment was with the assistant dean of the school, who could not have been more encouraging about the opportunities they had to offer. She was instantly easy to talk to. I shared my passions and desires for nursing and my views about the state of health care. They had multiple programs that included a nursing administration track, which was my area of interest. I felt the possibilities and got excited. Then suddenly I shot up out of the chair, panicked, and announced that I had no ability to pay.

She calmly replied, "What does your husband do?"

I said, "Theatre."

She smiled broadly and said, "Oh, there's money for you."

This kind of question would probably not be allowed today to avoid bias in applicant selection. But at that time my answer demonstrated economic need. The paths to my graduate education opened up. I was accepted into the school and a work-study program that covered my tuition and living expenses. I was assigned to assist Dean Palmer, the dean of the nursing school and a Florence Nightingale scholar. Palmer put me to work organizing and filing her mounds of Nightingale three-by-five index cards, each covered with her handwritten research notes. I was filled with Nightingale stories as I sorted those cards, making Nightingale's legacy vivid and real to me. On the other hand, my time spent reading the index cards slowed my productivity, which Dean Palmer pointed out routinely.

Graduate-level classes with smart, savvy nurses are always an education and entertaining. Listening to their work life experiences from school nursing, free health clinics, pediatrics, and public health opened my eyes wide. Topics covered the social, regulatory, political, and legal dimensions of nursing, medicalization of health care, male dominance, paternalism, ethics, and role struggles. The faculty threaded nursing theory, science, clinical advancements, and advanced practice roles through our work life experiences to illustrate their impact on our daily practice. I got swept up in the wonder of Martha Rogers's theory; it was a nursing framework that matched my worldview, although I never considered its application in the real world.

I bonded with several classmates, who became life friends. Tragically, one of our fellow students was murdered in her garage in our first year, not far from where I lived. Our class wondered how this could have happened to such a vibrant person and in her own home. She was a knowledgeable, strong leader in her professional community, job, and classes. I think of her every year when I hang the Christmas ornament on our family tree made by the underprivileged kids she worked with as a fundraiser. We had little information about her murder or her life outside what she talked about in class. Later in a local paper, it indicated that her husband was a suspect. I remember that we were all shocked that she could be a victim of a domestic murder; she was not the "victim type" in our view. We know much more now about domestic abuse and how there is no stereotypical victim type among its victims.

Nursing administration was my program track. To expand my perspective beyond nursing, I enrolled in two business seminars with master in business administration (MBA) students. I was struck by how much more of the real world we see as nurses compared to those in business, at least those in these business classes. One day, I took it upon myself to talk bluntly about male domination in health care and suppression of women's participation in organizational decision-making and in high leadership roles. I don't recall the words I used, but they must have been overpowering since my statements stopped the conversation, instead of advancing it. I remember the stunned expressions on their faces and the silence in the room once I stopped talking. I didn't see this as my problem, at the time. But eventually, I understood that it doesn't matter if you're right about something if you're not effective in communicating it.

Through school, I continued working in my community hospital. What I liked most about working in a community hospital level of critical care was that the patients were sick but not so sick that they were incapacitated. As a nurse, I could be there to help them and their families weave connections through the facts, feelings, and questions toward an understanding and meaning, so they could start to regain life stability. I loved that role.

There were many memorable cases in this beach community hospital where I felt I made a difference. There was the young mother whose seven-year-old daughter died of a head injury after falling off the Sunset Cliffs. After delivering the brain death diagnosis to the mother, the pulmonologist literally stood rigid in the hallway, staring straight ahead, stunned with his own emotions, as the mother sank slowly down to the ground sobbing, holding onto his body, nearly tearing off his lab coat. I ended up on the floor with the mother to try to comfort her. All of us were helpless. Another case involving drugs and a gunshot wound created quite a whirlwind. A stylish young woman in her twenties, upon gaining consciousness, decided in a flurry that she had to leave the unit against medical advice with a small-caliber bullet still lodged beneath her skull. Her goal was to retrieve her drug stash before the boyfriend could run off with it. She spoke coherently but shared no details with the police about how she got shot. It was assumed that it was a drug deal gone bad. The neurosurgeon was on his way in to take her to surgery. But she had other plans. The police couldn't intervene because she wouldn't cooperate with them. And neither could we; that bullet was not going to stop her. My discharge instructions were short and to the point: "get to a hospital after your mission is accomplished." I called her a cab, and away she went. And finally, there was the businessman with stock tips. He was a big, gregarious guy who heartily gave financial advice to all who entered his room. In the middle of having a serious heart attack, he announced the best stock market advice ever—buy stocks of the companies who make the products you love. To this day, David follows this advice—Starbucks, Costco, and Apple.

While I was holding on to caring moments, science and clinical complexity were advancing. This was during the time when adverse event data across the country were starting to paint an alarming picture—hospitals were killing patients. The pressure was on. Strict practice standards were becoming the norm, and nurses were in a steep learning curve to comply. I got swept up in one standardization in action incident when one of my patients extubated himself. He was being weaned off the ventilator that day, and I took his self-extubation as an opportunity to evaluate if he could breathe on his own before I called a physician.

In those few seconds, another nurse rushed in and exclaimed, "What are you doing? He needs to be reintubated."

It was not a situation to debate. All went well. A physician arrived and he was reintubated. I felt the loss of "wiggle room"—no time to pause. Standardization and risk-avoidance were becoming the hard rule. At the same time, I was finishing up my program coursework. It was good timing to explore other clinical arenas as I considered leadership opportunities.

# PART II

## GROWING MY NURSE LEADER SELF

# CHAPTER 4

# Finding My Place

Fortunately, my first official leadership position and new clinical specialty found me. It happened in my same community hospital where I had been working in critical care. The hospital had been recently acquired by a growing health care system in San Diego. One of the first moves this health care system undertook was to expand their rehabilitation services in my community hospital. In 1982, as I was finishing my MSN, I was offered an opportunity to develop and manage a new stroke rehabilitation unit. What a gift.

## Developing a Stroke Rehab Program

I had little knowledge of rehabilitation when I was offered this job, but after a bit of research, I realized that my clinical philosophy was in sync with rehabilitation's purpose and principles. Rehabilitation services are holistic and about teamwork and family integration in all aspects of care. Here I could learn more about helping people stabilize and rebuild their lives. The significance of me doing this work did not escape me, given my dad's devastating stroke at a young age. This was a perfect fit on many levels. I was blessed to work with an exemplary team of nurses, physicians and therapists. The teams' clinical expertise and interpersonal connections transformed patients' lives. My learning curve in both rehabilitation and leadership kept me stimulated and satisfied for many years.

Vernon Nickel was our rehabilitation medical director. He had recently moved from his world-renowned rehabilitation hospital in Los Angeles to do work in medical engineering as a member of the medical school faculty at the University of California San Diego. Vern was a big man with an unassuming presence as he casually walked the unit and departments daily, taking in everything. The only thing he didn't retain was people's names. One of the first things I learned from Vern was his view of rehabilitation nurses. He felt that nurses were the lynchpin to rehabilitation care, which was why he supported a nurse to run the program.

"Nurses are the orchestra leaders of rehabilitation, Pat. Go out there and conduct," he would say in our conversations.

Vern was an orthopedic surgeon and was known globally for his decades of work in rehabilitation and medical engineering. He had developed the halo device for stabilization of cervical spine fractures and other medical engineering advancements. Most importantly to me, Vern was an expert mentor. He stopped by my office almost daily. Vern listened as I talked him through my observations or issues of the day, and he would point out how my instincts and judgments were correct or not and why. These conversations were golden. My questions often prompted him to tell a story, which always had a point—how a good physician thinks or acts, what a good therapist is looking for, the problems or warning signs good nurses pick up on, etc. Vern loved telling stories about his experiences and life lessons. My husband, David, and I saw him a couple of times at David's theatre in Balboa Park, catching an evening show and enjoying the park. My confidence and clarity grew under his leadership. I knew he was special to me, but I didn't realize then just how rare a blessing he was. I never had that kind of relationship with a leader or mentor again.

The other person who benefited from Vern Nickel's wisdom and mentorship was David Simon. David was a young neurologist building his neurology practice in San Diego in the mid-'80s. He took over the medical directorship position of the stroke rehab program when Vern retired. David was drawn to rehab for the same philosophical reasons as I was. He too had studied anthropology and wanted to be a part of a holistic approach and teamwork. We had a good partnership. During the time he and I worked together, we were both mastering our leadership roles and parenting toddlers. We often laughed at ourselves behaving like responsible people at work, while at home we—and our spouses—were being outsmarted by our respective toddlers. David Simon later became affiliated with Deepak Chopra and was the cofounder and medical director of the Chopra Center for Well-being in the mid-'90s.

## How Our Family Grew

David and I didn't always know that we wanted to have kids. But once I started working fulltime, I wondered, *Is this all there is?* We had almost always been a family of three. Early in our relationship one summer in college, we got a puppy together without thinking it through. Not smart. He was the best dog ever; we named him James, after both of our fathers. When we proceeded to move apart as planned that fall, neither one of us would give up the puppy. So we stayed together. That probably says a lot about our relationship. Later in Ohio, we decided we would start having kids once we moved to San Diego.

The childbearing years showed us what loss of control feels like. There were heartbreaks and blessings all along the way—an unexpected pregnancy that ended in a premature stillbirth, followed by years of infertility, an adoption process that didn't get off the ground. Then we had a surprise pregnancy that produced a healthy premature baby, more infertility followed, and then a successful adoption—our second baby girl. In the end, it all happened just as it was supposed to.

We were thirty-two when our family expanded. Both of our daughters were born in San Diego – our oldest, a preemie, at University of California San Diego (UCSD) in 1983, and our youngest at Sharp Mary Birch Hospital in 1988 through an open adoption. Nurses played a special role in each birth. Our little preemie was born at thirty-one weeks weighing three pounds, "a rose," the resident called her. She was a grower for four weeks in their neonatal intensive care unit. Within those first few days of being there, the clinical nurse specialist (CNS) sheepishly approached David and me to ask if we would participate in a cardio pulmonary resuscitation (CPR) class and an interview. She was apologetic for the timing of this, but a film crew was coming to do a news segment on the importance of parents of preemies learning CPR to avert sudden infant death syndrome (SIDS). I remember thinking, *Oh dear, I didn't know there was a connection between SIDS and preemies.* UCSD was one of the first hospitals to include a CPR class in discharge education for preemie parents. I suspect that the CNS chose us—given David's theatre background—to guarantee that this important message would be delivered well in the interview for national television on *CBS Nightly News* with Dan Rather. We were still in a haze when the CNS asked us so we didn't catch the details about the CBS nightly news until right before it aired a month later. We were happy that we had agreed. We were able to give our families in Oklahoma a head's up so they could see the baby on TV in almost real time. This was way before the internet and smartphones. David's grandmother called him that night to say how pleased she was to see her namesake. She died in her sleep that night. We have cherished that video for thirty-five years now.

Five years later we adopted our youngest baby girl through an open adoption process. Open adoption was still new then. I had learned about open adoption and its important benefits in nursing school in Oklahoma many years earlier. Adoption agencies in San Diego in the '80s were not doing open adoption. To the rescue, a friend and attorney—the husband of one of my graduate school friends—knew of one attorney in San Diego who did open adoptions. That attorney made it all happen. As required, we submitted a grand family portfolio—full of pictures and stories. The birth parents then select parents to meet and interview based on the portfolios. David and I met the birth parents when they were three months pregnant.

Two months later, they met our four-year-old daughter, who promptly announced to the birth mother, "That baby inside of you is mine."

Out from the mouth of babes. We were speechless when we heard our daughter's statement. This was totally unprompted. We had been so careful in how we had introduced the adoption process to her in terms a four-year-old could understand. We were shocked that she could come out with such a direct statement.

Our little outspoken daughter stayed with our close friends—a psychiatrist and occupational therapist—thereafter during the subsequent times we met with the birth parents. The psychiatrist earnestly did anticipatory counseling with us through the process, trying to keep us realistic should the outcome be bad. But David never doubted that the adoption would work out, and he was right. I believe that it was our daughter and golden retriever who really sealed the deal. This experience does have its risks, but the rewards are magical. David and I were present during her delivery. David jumped in as the delivery coach, improvising with breathing exercises used by actors. I was the first to hold our baby girl. The whole situation was bittersweet and life changing. The birth parents kept her with them that first night at the hospital. The next morning, the nurses called us frantically because the birth parents had announced that they were packing up and taking the baby home. I assured the nurses that we were on our way, and yes, we were all taking our baby home at discharge. The expression on the nurses' faces when we walked into the hospital was profound relief. We knew from the beginning that it was important for a child to have the birth parents involved in his/her life, and so it has been for thirty years. We have all learned how to navigate an open adoption life.

## Back to Acute Care Nursing

Once our new baby girl arrived in 1988, I started looking for a new job. I wanted to return to acute care nursing in a leadership position. I had been in rehabilitation nursing for seven years, and the impact of the rapid changes in health care on nursing were calling me back. Patients were living longer, impacting how nursing care was delivered. I wanted to be a part of supporting and strengthening nurses and nursing in the midst of the expanding medicalization of health care. But my lack of current experience in acute care nursing became a barrier to a leadership position there. I reached out to a high-level nursing administrator in my health care system for direction. He advised that changing clinical fields in leadership required flexibility and willingness to take risks. The competition was already high; San Diego was becoming saturated with master-prepared nurse leaders. He connected me with a chief nursing officer (CNO) in Los Angeles, who was looking for a seasoned leader to help her turn her hospital around.

When I went to Los Angeles for an interview, I purposely avoided thinking about how disruptive this move would be for our family. However, I knew that David was behind me if the move was needed to advance my career. He was doing freelance directing by this time, which meant that he could live anywhere. The position was director of critical care and the emergency department in a small North Hollywood hospital. Right off, I was impressed with the

CNO; she had a PhD and was also the editor of *Nursing Economics* at the time. What a learning opportunity for me! She was the first nurse leader PhD I had met. She was smart, warm, and fun. I took the job, and my family and I moved to Los Angeles in 1989. It was a crash course in acute care nursing management. My CNO was loaded with health care knowledge and emotional intelligence. She had an organizational political ease that disarmed everyone— physicians, the executive team, and staff. I soaked up all the mentoring I could get. I was there for a year. I left after my CNO left. Fortunately, I had gotten the acute care leadership experience I needed to be more marketable. We moved back home to San Diego in 1990. Ironically, I landed a job at my original community hospital as director of acute care. The risk had paid off, although it was stressful for all. David and I were learning how to be our adventurous selves with children in tow.

## Who Am I?

It was becoming a mother of a baby girl that ushered me into therapy in 1983. Being a woman and a nurse, I knew male dominance and patriarchy existed, and I felt it in my marriage of ten years. David was an ongoing challenge for me when it came to dominance in our relationship. Let's just say that as an artistic type, cardiovascular surgeons had nothing over this guy. As a parent, I wanted to be a good role model for our daughter. And as a good wife, I needed to learn how to better communicate my emotions and to curb my reactivity. But to be honest, I wanted a therapist with credibility and authority to show David that it was him who needed to learn to communicate better and to show him that it was his behaviors that disrupted our relationship.

I started with the hospital's employee assistance program. Stress reduction was the first topic. I had taken up Transcendental Meditation (TM) when we first moved to San Diego. I figured if there was ever a life that required transcendence, it was being a nurse; TM helped. But I needed more after becoming a leader and a parent. TM had become hollow; I couldn't meditate my growing gut grip away. Initially David went to therapy with me, although there was "nothing wrong with me," he would say. He took to stress-reduction techniques right away and has used them to this day, he says. I think David's view of therapy was that he would focus on stress reduction and I would focus on me. And that's how it kind of played out in the early years of therapy. Basically, David saw nothing wrong in our relationship. "Everything is fine," was his line, as long as I didn't question or challenge him. My therapy assignment was to observe what triggered my angst and anger and try to use healthier communication techniques instead of overreacting. That's what I focused on. It was a start.

Within a year or so, I found a therapist who specialized in relationships. She was the real deal. I knew that with her, I had a chance to get to the bottom of what ailed our relationship. I continued to believe that David was the root cause of my emotional reactions, and if someone would just see that, I would be exonerated.

So after months of me telling her stories about how he had an anger thing and a dominant male thing, she said, "Well, let's bring him in."

*Yes, now!* I thought. David agreed to join me in a session with my new therapist. There we sat, the show down was finally going to happen, and I had someone on my side.

She said to him, "Pat tells me that you have an anger thing about women?"

He said, after a dramatic pause, "No, I don't have an anger thing about women."

She asked him a few more questions and then turned to me slowly and said, "Pat, he says that he doesn't have an anger thing about women."

I was stunned. *That's it? This is how we are going to leave this?* I thought. The therapist then led David and me in a conversation about anger management and communications and how to talk and listen to each other. The session was up. I made an appointment to return the following week, alone.

When David and I got to the car, our eyes locked over the top of the car while he unlocked the doors, and he said, smiling, "You thought you had me, didn't you?"

My thoughts flashed, and his words sunk in. All I could do was laugh out loud. He was right. It was a bit of a setup. We drove off laughing.

Over the following years, what this therapist helped me see was that even though my husband may need to dominate and resist being challenged, my first priority was to control me. There's no doubt that learning how to communicate better helped me feel better about myself and be a better role model as a mother. The arguments decreased by half-ish, and problem solving life's complex challenges together improved. And regarding David's growth? This therapist taught me two important lessons that apply to all people. Number one, the goal can never be to control others. And number two, no one can grow and change unless they choose to. Along with this, my self-awareness kept growing. Once I stopped identifying David as my problem, I started to see me more clearly. And that is the rest of the story.

# CHAPTER 5

# New Adventures

By 1992, we were off on another adventure that took us to Colorado. We had longed to move to Colorado when we lived there during summer jobs in college. My position at my San Diego community hospital was eliminated in 1991, and we had to make a choice. David was still freelancing, which took him away from home directing theatre and film several months per year. San Diego had become financially restricting; it was time for a house with more than two bedrooms. The vice president of nursing in a hospital in Colorado often came to San Diego to sail. She had read an article in a local paper about the downsizing of San Diego hospitals. And so she ran a classified ad for a director of medical surgical services figuring that there were seasoned nurse leaders in southern California who would love to come to Colorado. She was right. I accepted the job. David and I were thrilled. What a perfect place to raise our girls. They were ages nine and four when we moved.

David has a saying, "Live where others want to vacation."

Well, we certainly achieved that with this move. San Diego was spectacular, and the Black Forest in Colorado was equal. We were blessed once again. The Black Forest is just north of Colorado Springs at an altitude of seventy-three hundred feet. David found and bought our new house when he took a separate trip to scout the area after I accepted the job. We now had a three-bedroom house on two and a half acres of horse property in a community with eighty acres of common land where the girls could run and play freely. It was ideal by David's and my standards, but only he had seen it when he bought it before we moved.

When I had started working in Colorado and had the girls with me, we got access to the house. David was back in San Diego packing up for the final move. That first drive out to the Black Forest to see our new home was long and full of anticipation. Our oldest daughter was already going through the expected adjustments of a new school and finding new friends. Our little one was taking the move in stride. That first drive seemed like an eternity.

Both girls piped up with comments as we drove, "Where is it? Are we there yet? There's nothing out here. Really, this far?"

Thankfully, upon arrival to the house, the girls were won over by their separate bedrooms. The property was breathtaking, covered with Ponderosa pines and fresh snow. The drive got shorter the more often we drove it. It's amazing how easy it is to adjust when it's beautiful. The daily drive to work became a motion meditation along the front range of the Rocky Mountains with Pikes Peak jetting up out of the high plains to fourteen thousand feet. Stunning every day. And when the girls were with me, the drives provided quality time together.

## A Happy, Growing Organization

My new hospital was an established, city-owned, nonprofit, community hospital. It was a stand-alone organization, and the leaders were eager to make it a major player in the Colorado health care market. It felt like an adolescent organization. We were perpetually growing and changing into the next thing. The emergency department grew into the busiest in the state, driven by population growth and distribution of hospitals in the area. Other volume contributors were the city's drug and gang growth over the years due to the drug trafficking up and down the Interstate 25 corridor between Mexico to Canada, and its proximity to a large army base south of the city. Active outdoor lifestyles and the Olympic Training Center fed the sports medicine and orthopedic services. In addition, the high altitude triggers heart and lung illnesses and premature births. It was a busy place. The physicians were dedicated and progressive; it felt like cowboy medicine all over again. It was a good place for trauma surgeons to use their skills upon returning from the Gulf War. The administrative leaders were successful businessmen. The nursing leaders were independent and smart. High values were at the core of the organization's culture. It always felt like we were on the right side in health care's trajectory. It was a happy place to learn and grow.

# CHAPTER 6

# Finding Caring

One of the most professionally enlightening endeavors my new hospital provided was our involvement in the *Colorado Differentiated Practice Model* research project (Levi, Montgomery, and Hurd 1994).[5] Right after I arrived in 1992, I knew I was in the right place when I learned that the nursing leaders had agreed to participate in this three million–dollar statewide research project sponsored by the Colorado Trust. It was exciting to be exposed to such a large-scale nursing research project. This was nursing science in the making. The researchers who oversaw this project were protégés of Jean Watson, a nurse theorist from the University of Colorado I had learned about in graduate school.

The *Colorado Differentiated Practice Model* study grew out of the need to define a nursing care delivery model that would improve patient outcomes and satisfy nurses by putting the right nurse in the right job based on his/her education—licensed practical nurse, associate degree nurse, baccalaureate nurse, masters nurse, and doctorate nurse—and experience level. The Colorado Trust's interest was the impending quality and financial demands of health care reform and the nursing shortage. The research studied two hundred nurses of five different education levels in diverse health care settings across Colorado, and their relationships across patient quality outcomes (using nurse-sensitive indicators), patient satisfaction, resource utilization, and nurse satisfaction. I was proud to be a part of this; four of my medical surgical units were involved. The intrigue for me was the question, "Does authentic caring vary by nurses' education levels?" There is the assumption that patient satisfaction is higher when care is provided by baccalaureate nurses related to their expanded social science and humanities education. The results of the study did not demonstrate conclusive support of a differentiated practice model. However, there was evidence of a consistent association between baccalaureate preparation and RN practice outcomes.

During this project and in the following year in the mid-'90s I learned more about Jean Watson's human caring theory, processes, and caring leadership in other hospitals as we traveled across the country to present the study findings at conferences. I was filled with the promise of this growing caring science and practices. But it all stopped in our hospital when the research ended, and soon after throughout nursing. What followed was the surge in evidence-based practice standards. No longer was there interest in the impact of different levels of nursing education. The focus turned to hard science; every nurse was expected to follow practice standards in the same way, regardless of education levels. And in the midst of this, caring got sidelined.

# PART III

## BEING BLINDED

# CHAPTER 7

# Becoming Good

*Good To Great* by Jim Collins came out in 2001. This was an iconic book about the importance of organizational culture. It provided a roadmap for organizations to reach greatness. My hospital saw this as its destiny. I'm not sure the leadership team knew what becoming great meant for our organization. As the book points out, the key thing that makes organizations great is having one goal clearly understood by all (Collins 2001,116).[6] At this hospital, the physicians thought they were already great. I think we in the nursing department thought that we were just a few steps away from greatness. And the administrators were just waiting for the great money to roll in. Our main goal was to harness quality care in our city's growing market. We were riding the white water rapids of health care's rising science, technology, and reform in a middle-American city being redefined by its shifting social demographics. But at the core of our efforts was the heart of the organization. How we all loved this organization, its people, its values, and what it stood for—a city-owned hospital doing the right things for its community. It was an organization with a civic mission. And that's what we all rallied around.

As nurse leaders, our love and commitment to nursing and this organization was the glue of our working relationships with each other. The nursing service was the moral standard bearer and was strong clinically, known for its advanced nursing competencies, education, and training—so much so that the physicians complained that the nurses ran the hospital. In many ways nursing held the keys to the kingdom. Our nursing leadership team was smart, caring, well-intentioned, visionary, and committed to the mission of the hospital. We soldiered on doing all the things that other health care organizations do to be great, which for nursing meant shared governance, a professional practice model, a clinical advancement program, and a care delivery model, all designed to point us in the direction of Magnet Recognition standards.[7] We were a productive team. Together, we developed, mentored, and built teams, towers, and hospitals; expanding our 240-bed single hospital into a 670-bed three-hospital system over a fifteen-year period.

*Good to Great* was really about people and their willingness to face truths. And therein lies the challenge for many organizations. Ours was an organization not inclined to turn itself inside out to confront the brutal facts. It was hierarchical, steeped in history and stories of the past. As we grew, our bandwidth was maxed out; we didn't look up long enough to see ourselves in a mirror. One of the morals of *Good To Great* was that being good is the enemy of achieving greatness.[6] All in all, our organization was good.

## A Pediatrician's Office

As established earlier, respect is important within a family, and good communication skills help us express our truths in respectful ways. One of the best books on how to get to truths and communication is *How to Talk So Kids Will Listen and Listen So Kids Will Talk* by Adele Faber and Elaine Mazlish. I was guided to this parenting book when our oldest was three. To this day, it is one of my best parenting and leadership books, but I didn't figure the leadership part out for many more years. The three parenting lessons in the first nine pages had a huge impact on me: 1. Listen for the feelings. 2. Accept the feelings; never deny how the child says they're feeling. 3. Help the child give their feelings a name (Faber and Mazlish 2012 edition,1–46).[8] From there we as parents will get better cooperation, find the best corrections, encourage autonomy, learn how to praise, and more. The first three steps alone resolved the issues 90 percent of the time.

It worked wonders with our oldest daughter when she was in her terrible threes. This was a child who screamed so loud in a pediatrician's office once, we were asked to leave. It was a routine wellness appointment. Both David and I were there because these were important developmental evaluations for post-preemies. Not until we got to the exam room did we learn that she was afraid of going to the doctor. That's when she started bellowing at the top of her lungs. We were both caught off guard. We wanted to take her and flee. I remembered the book. I started asking her questions versus telling her to stop crying, which I desperately wanted to do. Then the pediatrician indicated that we needed to take it out of the room by popping his head in the door, with his stethoscope in one ear and holding the other earpiece away from his head, and glancing back at the other exam room, where he was obviously trying to listen to heart and lung sounds.

David was steaming. "Oh great, we're being kicked out of a pediatrician's office."

He was right—we were. I directed both David and our daughter out of the office to take a walk. I told the receptionist to hold the room and that we would be right back. As we walked around the block, we listened to her story, through her sobs. She was afraid that she was going to be put to sleep, as our sick dog had been the week before. As she got the story out, she settled down and stopped crying. Once we reentered the exam room, the pediatrician sat on the floor across the room from her, and we cryptically told him the basics about our dog. Slowly he was able to complete the developmental evaluation. His diagnosis: a normal, healthy three-year-old. From there, I started listening to connect her feelings to her behaviors and to see better how she saw her world in those moments of anger and terror. This got us through that stage and the following years, but life kept on rolling.

## Some Flip Charts

Moving to Colorado had its ups and downs. The intersection of our careers and family life cycles challenged David and me. When the gears grind, the sounds get ugly. The girls were nine and four when we moved there in 1992, and adolescence seemed to follow quickly. Through the mid-'90s, David traveled with his work a lot, and I was consumed in mine. Plus my mom died in 1995, which triggered lots of memory processing about our relationship during these years that added to my family ups and downs.

When David was away, the girls and I had a routine. It involved the usual stuff—driving to and from daycare, then catching the school bus, and always trying to get to work on time. As the girls got older, my expectations of their self-management heightened, and I became more reactive when they didn't meet my expectations. I would get upset when they were not ready in time to leave in the mornings or when they had not finished their homework and chores timely in the evenings. When I got too loud and demanding, they pulled away from me, and then I would self-correct. The girls and I stumbled along in this cycle for quite a while, until I woke up to signs of deeper trouble in our relationships.

By the time they were thirteen and eight, in 1996, my listening skills had broken down. I knew I had to find new ways of communicating with my older daughter to understand the real issues that were distancing us. She was starting to lash out at me with mean statements. I knew she needed me to hear her, but she wouldn't share in a normal conversation. At one point she locked herself in the closet out of protest over something. She was showing me that our connection was really broken.

I had learned how to flow-chart processes at work. It was a great way to bring people together to identify and improve issues. And my family needed improving. So one weekend afternoon, I got out an easel that I had borrowed from work, a big flip chart, and colored markers, which I knew would intrigue our eight-year-old. David was away, so I was winging it on my own. I introduced them to the goal, which was to get all of our issues onto the flip pages. Then we each would talk about them and figure out how to make them better. Nope, no one was impressed. These two girls were not willing to participate. I was stumped. So I started talking and drawing how I was feeling, with circles, boxes, and arrows going every which way. Still no reaction. Then I started stating what they might be thinking and feeling. My speculations had to be honest to make this authentic for them. This was hard for me, but it opened the door. My thirteen-year-old was not going to let me be her voice. Finally she started voicing her truths, going right to the tender spots. It's widely accepted that adolescents' honesty can shake anyone's foundation. It was my job to be quiet and listen. I learned a lot. My younger daughter piped up with a few observations and then said, "Are we done yet?" It was priceless, those girls sitting on the floor telling me their thoughts, feelings, and truths, and me writing and drawing flow diagrams without comment or judgment, just soaking it in. The conclusions were the following:

- We three would be supportive and respectful (my older daughter's word) of each other.
- I was not to raise my voice.
- Homework would be completed before phone calls, play, or television.
- We would have an outing together every Wednesday evening.
- If the girls were not ready to leave in the morning when I got in the car, they would be left behind. (I don't think that ever happened.)

- We would have more hugging and cuddling time.
- As a follow-up, we would evaluate how well we were keeping our promises.

This process worked. I saw what they saw. It was painful. Our relationships shifted for the better from that day on. Relief. As Farber and Mazlish's book teaches, what you hear when you listen are the true feelings. I was listening.

## My Red Cape

My first clue that my firewall between work and home had broken down was when a new member of our nursing leadership team said, "Good morning, Pat. How are you? Is your red cape on or off today?"

This greeting occurred as I was walking into the boardroom where we had our weekly administrative meeting. I and others laughed; her delivery was quite funny. At first, I took the red cape comment as a description of my decisive manner and language; then I realized that it was not so positive. Internally I kicked into ego protection, and then I wondered, what did it mean and how real was it?

Soon after, I found out that it was very real. Two leaders on my management team came to me to say that they dreaded our weekly division meetings. They said that they left these meetings feeling defeated and exhausted every week from the pressures and demands I wielded. My self-image as a trusted leader disintegrated. After the pain and embarrassment passed, I knew their honesty was a gift, but it took time to see clearly.

I had not realized how uncertain I felt about the work changes happening around me until these conversations. We had been in the midst of organizational structure and role changes for several years, along with mounting workloads. Up until then, I had been blinded by my defensive self-confidence. One day while walking down the long hallway to my office, I heard a "voice" criticizing my behavior after a meeting. The hallway was empty; it was just me. There I was all dressed up in my executive best—red suit, white lace–collared blouse, pearls, shiny black heels, and big hair—listening to this ranting voice: "That was a dumb statement. You should have said …" It was an ugly voice; it had a twisted face, like a child's face when they are fearfully saying hurtful things to another. This voice was mine. The deeper I got into my self-help books, the more I acknowledged my self-doubt in my job performance. This felt new, and it was not just unsettling; it was destabilizing. I soon learned that self-doubt goes hand-in-hand with self-awareness, until you gain perspective. This was not an easy process, but I had to keep going.

Around this time, the early 2000s, our oldest started driving and was pushing for more independence. I wanted to handle this well, so I decided it was time to get back into therapy. Right away, the therapist suggested family therapy to work on conflict resolution. What a gift. We went through several family sessions focusing on control and letting go. In one session, our oldest daughter, then sixteen, told David that she felt like she had lost her best friend when he started traveled with work and when they started arguing a lot. That was real and tearful. From there, our therapist talked about feelings of fear and vulnerability associated with loss of control. For David it was losing control of his little girls, as they were growing more independent. For me, it was feeling loss of control at work.

The therapist helped me see the ins and outs of my fears and control at work. After one afternoon session alone with the therapist where he and I worked through the red cape statement and the stress I had caused my managers, I sat in the car and cried until relief came. What I had to accept was that when truth and self-awareness come, another set of issues set in: guilt, shame, and vulnerability—feelings that I had spent a lifetime avoiding. I knew they were there, but I had not allowed them in. Acting like I was right all the time was hard work, and learning to accept that I wasn't right became even harder work for a while. The ironies of self-management were upon me. The good news was I had control of my destiny on a level that I had never imagined possible. The bad news was I had control of my destiny on a level that I had never imagined possible. This new perspective was freeing and opened deeper paths for growth in all of my relationships at work and at home.

Self-help books were a constant source of emotional growth and health. In the mid-'90s, I read, made notes, and then listened repeatedly to three iconic works during my daily commute to and from work along the eastern slope of the Pikes Peak region: Scott Peck's *The Road Less Traveled*, Andrew Weil's *Spontaneous Healing*, and Wayne Dyer's *Real Magic*. Evidence of Eastern philosophies and spiritual traditions transforming our Western ways was in full swing. These health practices were entering our daily routines, and mind-body science and lifestyle medicine were starting to redirect modern medicine. My growing self-awareness, observations, and conversations with others made it clear that I was not the only middle-aged nurse, leader, wife, and mother going through relationship and work challenges and revelations. I was certain that my social and emotional struggles were not unique to me. This made me wonder how these learnings could help nursing and nurses individually and collectively. How was nursing science integrating holistic and self-help practices and mind-body medicine? By 1999, it was time to return to school. Once again, when in doubt, go back to school.

The University of Colorado (CU) was right up the road in Denver. Finally I could learn more about Jean Watson's caring theory and processes. I was looking for solutions and an infusion of hope for me as a nurse leader and for nurses working in the health care industry. What I learned was much more. Watson did indeed understand the social, scientific, and ethical waves of change and their impact on nursing. Her work was designed to take us beyond what existed.

# Chapter 8

# School Was My Refuge

Through the early 2000s, I completed the foundation courses in the doctorate in philosophy (PhD) program at the CU Denver Health Science Center, College of Nursing. Nursing's connections with mind-body spirit science spun me around. One afternoon my younger daughter, twelve years old then, and I were driving to pick up her ice skates, and I was listening to a National Public Radio series recording of Bill Moyer's interviews with neuroscientists, *Healing and the Mind* (1993).[9] It was revealing the mind's impact on the body's health and healing as we rode along.

At one point Moyer stated, "You mean to tell me that the mind is in every cell of our body?"

I almost ran off the road. "Did you hear that?" I exclaimed to my daughter.

She couldn't help but hear it. At that point I had her start taking notes as we listened—there were no handy smartphones back then. That was her life through those years, listening to my verbal downloads of what I was learning when I was excited or inspired. She is now attending a nursing PhD program, so this must have triggered a connection along the way. Mind and health topics breathed new life into nursing and humanity for me. Human connection is nursing's arena. School became my refuge from the real world.

The real world was a lot to handle; I and my fellow nurse leaders at work were consumed with the competing demands of growth and expansion, evidence-based practice, scaling up quality improvements, rolling out the electronic medical record, and building a new tower and then a new hospital. Regarding caring, we did the standard integration of Watson's caring theory into our professional practice model and programs, but nothing beyond that.

The reality was that even though I was studying caring theory in school and learning caring processes in Watson's caring courses, I didn't have an overwhelming drive to implement an authentic caring expansion plan in my organization, mainly because I didn't see a path. I saw authentic caring practices and caring consciousness cultivation as a personal journey for each nurse to be done on their own through self-care practices. I didn't understand how nurse leaders could impact each nurse's personal journey. And the idea of an organizational scope of caring based on caring theory and science seemed wholly unrealistic given the demands of our organizational workloads. The closest my organization came to implementing a caring practice model to support nurses in their caring practices was bringing in consultants from a caring relationship program, twice. Each time they provided onsite workshops, first with our nurse leaders at an annual retreat, and years later the consultants returned to do workshops with our charge nurses and shared governance councils. The focus of the latter was on development of caring interventions and processes for the direct caregivers. The expectation of the nurse leaders remained the same: be bearers of the caring philosophy, nothing else.

# CHAPTER 9

# Caring—Health Care Industry Style

The pace of health care changes escalated as we entered the new century. The common knowledge was there were more changes occurring in the last five years of the '90s than in all time. This aptly described what was going on in hospitals. So when Emmett Murphy, author of *Leadership IQ in Hospitals*,[10] proclaimed at a VHA (Voluntary Hospitals of America) Leadership Conference in 2000 that health care was the single most complex industry there was—over aeronautics, space, government—and that acute care nurse leaders had the single most complex job over all other jobs, I shot my hand up and exclaimed, "Amen." Finally, there was an explanation for the stress levels hospital nurse leaders were living through on a daily basis.

## When Theme-Park Magic Came to Town

Along with the science and technological advances, the spotlight had shifted to nurses' caring performance in the early 2000s. The race within the hospital industry to produce high customer satisfaction scores was on. Nationwide aggregate measurements for comparisons of patient satisfaction became available and would be monetized in the future. This was the beginning of clinicians being evaluated by consumers on a grand scale and the insurers using data to hold the health care industry accountable.

Patients having a voice is a good thing. Up until then, patients had no voice; we in the health care professions had dictated what health care was to look like for patients. I remember the days of passing meds with the attitude of "I know what is best for you." These days were gone. We had to adjust to patients having a voice. The satisfaction scores were real and would be driving reimbursement.

So when Fred Lee presented his theme-park magic principles, the health care industry was ready to listen. He presented at my hospital's 2006 annual leadership retreat, and I fell for its shiny goodness just like I did the first time I went to the iconic theme park as a kid. Lee presented from his book, *If Disney Ran Your Hospital*.[11] All four hundred–plus leaders from my organization heard how caring can feel like magic. He presented caring as an attitude, a desire to attend to patients' comfort needs and to make sure patients felt special. The chief-suite and all department heads saw this as nursing's responsibility. We nurse leaders initially took the magical focus as a gift because it felt like recognition and support. (Note—Lee's parallels between theme parks and health care were based on the knowledge he had picked up from the four nurses in his family.) Within a year, this magical idea rolled into a hospitality program, which gave legs to our customer satisfaction initiatives as part of our organizational pillars of excellence. Soon there were scripts engaging all staff in patient satisfaction—response scripts, hallway etiquette, rounding programs.

These scripted, formulaic programs marked a turning point in caring within the health care industry. Monetization of caring has driven the stakes higher and puts pressure on nurses to create the best caring experience possible for patients. The meaning of caring took on a different charge once the health care industry leaders took an interest in caring as a direct way to raise patient satisfaction scores and reimbursement. As scripted formulaic programs proliferated, we got scripts on how to greet patients, how to give directions, how to close conversations, etc. These programs are well intentioned and do help provide a baseline standard for caring cultures across organizations. But these programs can come at a price.

Problems arise when scripted programs set standards for nurse caring initiatives on two levels: 1. The programs imply that these are high-level standards for nursing care. 2. The programs do not acknowledge or build on nurses' existing authentic caring practices. These messages create confusion and resistance among nurses. I know from experience that nurse leaders can get caught between the promotion of and nurses' resistance to scripted programs. These programs have a support role in organizations, but not as the end game of nurse caring. Scripted programs rise out of a vacuum in the health care industry left by nurse leadership at large not giving a clear and consistent voice to high-level caring as defined in caring science and as demonstrated by nurses' existing authentic caring. Scripted caring programs have distanced us as nurse leaders from nurses and our caring essence.

## The Business of Caring

There was a trend in the '90s, where many nurse leaders went through MBA programs for their graduate education. I always thought that was unfortunate; they missed out on studying the history and growth of nursing science. But on the other hand, business practices are important in the health care industry, so I understood it as a career strategy. MBA or not, financial acumen and organizational strategies are necessary skills for all leaders.

It was impossible to escape the business world mindset as a leader in hospitals. The fact is that nurse leaders are wedged between two major forces—medicine and business—making it easy to lose one's sense of nursing identity and integrity, philosophically and practically. The overarching facts are: Medicine is in the business of saving lives and improving lives. Health care is in the business of providing medical services in caring organizations. Nursing balances all of these—saving lives, improving lives, and caring. It is nurses who attend to patients' deep, human caring needs associated with suffering and healing in vulnerable moments. But that's not what the health care industry supports and what nursing leadership resembles. Being a nurse leader in the health care industry can dull one's sensibilities, largely related to the high demands of

—medicine, business, and technology and the low reward ratio in authentic caring in organizations. It is experiencing the essence of nursing in authentic caring that keeps us in the game, nurses and nurse leaders alike. This is where meaning and purpose are derived in nursing.

The gap between business and caring turns into a chasm the further up the leadership ladder a nurse goes. And once there, that chasm seems insurmountable and wholly unrealistic to fill for nurse leaders. Nurse leader competencies shift to business and technology. Leadership of caring morphs into structures and measurements and becomes less authentic. I was one of many well-intentioned leaders who did not have the impact on caring practices I longed to achieve because I did not see realistic options amid the forces around me and the responsibilities in front of me.

## The Power of Team

In the eight years following the red cape statement and my managers waving the stress flag, my management team became my growing ground. Their honesty with me was a pivot point in my leadership. My self-awareness intensified as I took advantage of the groundswell of wellness books and programs. Emotional intelligence entering the leadership literature added to my self-growth toolbox. At work, to change the experience of our meetings, I started using flip chart papers on the walls in every meeting to keep me more centered and focused on team participation around the agenda; these flip pages became our minutes.

I was in school at CU during these years, and the rest of my management team were in different stages of their masters. They adopted the "when in doubt, go back to school" life philosophy. We shared our school learnings and self-discoveries— dominated by evidence-based practice, quality improvement projects, and technology. Here I shared caring science and my DNP research, which was on self-care practices and caring efficacy. We lived the importance of self-development and wellness as a leader. This is the one thing I knew for certain: nurse leaders had to be on a lifelong self-care learning path to survive and thrive. My team and I bonded and grew around that.

# CHAPTER 10

# Leaving Colorado

Leaving Colorado happened slowly and suddenly. My family celebrated a triple graduation in 2006. I graduated from CU Denver with my DNP, our older daughter graduated from CU Boulder, and our younger daughter from high school. By 2008, the girls were on paths taking them away from Colorado. Our oldest moved to Brooklyn to pursue art in 2007, and our younger was heading to Africa in the Peace Corps in 2010 as soon as she graduated from CU Boulder. During these years of the girls' high school and college, David worked in Aspen, Colorado, as an artistic theatre director. The four of us drove all over the state those years keeping up with sports, theatre, and college events.

## ⟩ I Had to Be Kicked Out

Organizational changes at my hospital were a constant. The long-tenured executives were replaced one by one with leaders from within as they retired until the positions gave way to new faces from the outside. Several of my nurse leader colleagues moved on for their careers and adventures, and others retired. The new executive team hired a new CNO in 2008; her assignment was to challenge our status quo.

After an assessment and reorganization of the nursing services, the new CNO said to me, "What are you still doing here? You need to be a CNO."

Advice from an outsider I respected released me—from what I'm not sure. It was time for me to move on—past time. New adventure intrigue quickly set in. David was supportive of my new possibilities, although at first he was determined to stay in Colorado.

The seventeen years in Colorado from1992 to 2009 were transformative. I grew with my organization as it expanded from a single hospital to a three-hospital system. My initial position as director of four medical-surgical units evolved into one over the acute care services for the system—the adult medical and surgical units, patient flow management, the hospitalist's care management team, a palliative care team, the ethics committee, and care management. One dear Colorado coworker wrote me, "You and yours are part of my fabric." My fabric is full of the wonder of Colorado and those dear people.

## It's Cold in Colorado

I had done some math. We lived at an altitude of seventy-three hundred feet. The growing season in the Black Forest is about two months per year. I had gotten into gardening and xeriscaping in Colorado as the girls grew older and David was away in Aspen. The math went like this: If I lived thirty more years and had only two months of gardening in warm weather each year, that is the equivalent of just five more years of being warm outdoors. Aging is one thing, but facing such a short amount of time in warmth was a reality I could not accept. Our yard was beautifully expansive and natural. It gave me a creative outlet in nature. I felt one with nature and God when I was in our yard with my dog and best buddy, Poggiolo. I wanted more time outside.

My CNO job search was wide open. David and I accepted that my next job could take me out of state. My main priority was to find a hospital with the right leadership team where I could grow and learn. I could work anywhere really. Recruiters matched me with organizations that were small and on a growth trajectory. As I started interviewing for my CNO job, Colorado's September snow guided me to look at warm-weather locations. These snows were bittersweet, stunningly peaceful, but always marking the end of gardening for the year. So I chose to focus on southern California, where the days are warm and the nights are cool, where our girls were born and where David and I became grownups.

## God's Country

Our years in Colorado gave the girls a full appreciation for open spaces, hiking, and camping; they became avid skiers, boarders, and backpackers. After adventuring hither and yon, they both now live in California. They visit Colorado often and have properly introduced their life partners to outdoor adventures that only the Colorado Rocky Mountains can offer. Colorado is certainly God's country. It was here that nature ushered me into deep spiritual growth. Being raised Catholic, David and I were familiar with the notion of majesty, but there is no majestic spirit like the Rocky Mountains. I am forever thankful for this spiritual place.

## PART IV

# BECOMING MY AUTHENTIC SELF

# CHAPTER 11

# I Landed in Corporate Health Care

So it was. I became a CNO and landed a job with a dream team. It was with a multihospital system, which was my goal after working in a stand-alone hospital where it felt like everything had to be created from scratch. My first interview was with the chief executive officer (CEO) and chief operating officer (COO) by phone. It was a conversation mainly about nursing and caring, filled with ease and laughter, and ended with, "Can you start tomorrow?"

It was an exhilarating and transforming five years from 2010 to 2015. Upon arrival, they were finalizing the construction of a beautiful five-story, 157-bed hospital with single rooms, wide hallways, windows ceiling to floor, and views all around. It was designed with future growth in mind. It was ten years in the making—mainly because it was positioned on the San Andreas fault line. After a year of preparations, four "day in a life" hospital-opening exercises, and several opening postponements, the grand opening finally happened. The move involved rotating caravans of ambulances transporting patients and staff from the old hospital to the new, with a parade of news agencies and cameras along the way. It was a grand day.

## My Ideal Team

What really stood out in this job was the executive team in those first two years; together we "moved mountains" and had fun doing it. The executives were smart, happy, authentic, and most of all caring. The CEO called people by name—staff, physicians, and community—and often knew about their family lives. He focused on building relationships and business development. He left the operations to us. The nurses trusted him, and by association they trusted me and the other executive leaders. He rarely missed a thing about what was going on; that was evident in his observations and questions.

The five years were a whirlwind. After the opening year, year two was adjusting to double patient volumes, rapid system corrections, and staffing and recruitment. In year three we implemented an integrated electronic medical record, big bang style. My last two years there involved reorganizing and stabilizing to advance quality practices and outcomes, which brought us statewide recognition for quality indicators. It was exhilarating and heart-wrenching at the same time because it was never enough—for the patients backed up in the emergency department waiting room, for the staff whose raises didn't come timely, for staffing cuts that required adjustments, etc. The advancements were always in the beginning stages, and that makes organizational dynamics fragile in any situation.

I had always known that being a CNO had added challenges, but I hadn't expected it to be an opportunity to transform myself. I was lucky to share my wellness and caring consciousness journey with a peer on the executive team. Part of my leadership challenge was being comfortable in vulnerability and shedding my need for self-protection. With her, I could do this. I explored caring science as a way of leading. She knew nothing about caring science but had an expanding worldview and wellness consciousness. We weathered the ups and downs together during my five years there. I recommend having at least one simpatico relationship in any inward journey. My favorite connection with her was learning and laughing at ourselves each time we "fell in the arena" (Brown, 2012).[12] Well, maybe I fell more often and had more to laugh about than she did.

## Being a Hot Mess in Corporate America

This hospital was part of a for-profit health care corporation that had multiple community hospitals across the country. Ready access to the CNOs at the other hospitals within the organization as well as clinical experts in the corporate offices was another highlight of the job. These nurse leaders provided a built-in support network of knowledge, wisdom workers. The corporate clinical leaders kept us focused and productive. The collective goal was to develop nursing organizational programs and a nursing infrastructure across all hospitals. During this time, we worked on a professional practice model, clinical nurse advancement program, frontline nurse leadership program, quality elements for the electronic medical record, and quality projects. Each CNO was to customize the programs in their hospital with staff participation. A strong sense of commitment to all of our patients, nurses, and communities united us.

On the local level, I experienced corporate politics up close after we opened the new hospital. Patriarchy and money drove corporate decisions and communications. The CEO who had hired me left within two years of my being there, and another CEO came and went after three months. The COO filled in until the next CEO came. As the pressures from the Value-Based Purchasing Program[13] rose across the health care industry, ill will toward the CNOs escalated. At one of our CNO leadership conferences, a corporate executive stood up in front of us and stated, "Maybe we have the wrong CNOs," when talking about nursing care and patient satisfaction. I remember that I responded to his comment with an explanation about how caring impacts satisfaction. Not helpful.

Job security for CNOs is often tenuous, especially in this organization. It was unsettling on the occasions when one of the CNOs left suddenly. Looking back, the first clue that my job could be at risk was when the last CEO I worked with there stated, "The staff doesn't see you as part of the executive team, Pat." This was on a day after he had made hospital rounds within the first year of his arrival. I remember being surprised by the CEO's statement. I asked a question or two. He remained vague. I didn't know if this was a test of loyalty or if he didn't understand the facets of the nurse leader position. This is one of the perils characteristic of the nurse leader role on the executive level. We are often perceived as belonging to "the other side," depending on whom we are with. Are we on the side of nursing, on the side of medicine or administration? Until then, I had achieved being seen as both a nurse leader and an executive team player. The camaraderie within our team was palpable. Managing up is what we did. From there, I set up weekly meetings with him to review my role and contributions in the quality and satisfaction initiatives going on throughout the hospital. The meetings rarely happened.

A couple of years later, another statement surfaced casting doubt on my team effectiveness. It was on a conference call with a top corporate executive to get the preliminary impressions of an onsite labor union assessment. At the time of the impromptu conference call, several of us hurriedly gathered into the human resource director's office to sit in on the call. While waiting, we multitasked using hand signals to each other. On the call were the corporate executive, the union assessor, our human resources director, and our local executive team. It was just another conference call, until the assessor started to review her findings. She had met with various staff and asked them to rank order the administrative staff for level of leadership influence and credibility. I was ranked last. *Whoa, that can't be right*, I thought. I planned to get more details from the assessor after the call. Then suddenly the implications of this ranking registered when I heard the silence among those on the call and in the room. The assessor quickly made clear that she was still meeting with staff, and that there was more to come. And there was more to come. It turned out that the information she reported had not come from nurses or nursing departments. But the damage was done. Sometimes these kinds of misanalyses can weather storms, but not in a high-blame environment.

Now don't get me wrong, I had self-inflicted my share of corporate wounds—a couple of times. My level of emotional intelligence was progressing, but not enough to exhibit consistent political correctness. Sitting through lengthy presentations by corporate leaders targeting the CNOs was hard to take sometimes without a counter comment. One of my fellow CNOs aptly called my response a "hot mess" after one of those presentations. This was after I had shot up out of the chair and spoke in defense of the CNOs to the corporate quality efficiency leader who charged that the efficiency issues in the organization rested on the CNOs. That was the corporate line, and I took the bait. It was not my best hour and certainly dried the target ink on my back.

# CHAPTER 12

# Focusing on What Matters

I kept thinking that if the corporate politics could just settle down, I could start doing more meaningful work that would lend to professional development and morale. We CNOs had adopted Watson as our theorist as part of our professional practice model for all hospitals with the goal to implement. The CNOs had a vision for nursing despite the pressures. We plowed through our project meetings with blinders on, never losing hope for the positive impact nursing could have across the corporation if we were successful.

In year four of my CNO position, my hospital's nursing sensitive indicators, core measures, and readmission rates reached and exceeded state and national standards. Although this was thrilling, it couldn't sustain without a nursing infrastructure for staff development and participation. We needed to get more nurses involved in clinical improvement initiatives and develop their project and leadership skills. We launched three programs as building blocks toward a shared decision-making infrastructure where nurses could learn and lead: nurse handoff communication model, staffing committee, nurse advancement program. After a year of hard work, a team of nurses and the education and quality departments launched a successful hospital-wide bedside report program using the electronic record for all shift and department handoffs. This felt like space age progress at the time.

## Queries about Meaning

While expending time and energy to erect our nursing infrastructure, something happened that caused my leadership lens to flash open. I had often asked nurses questions about meaning in their practice in classes I taught. *How many days this week have you experienced meaning in your job?* As a leader, the purpose of the question was to identify how nurses were feeling about their practice in our hospital. The answers were pretty consistent. I got used to hearing the response of between zero and one day per week. And then suddenly I noticed bewildered expressions across the faces of the nurses as they heard the question for the first time. I could see that they hadn't thought of their work in this way for a while, as if they were being reminded that their work once had meaning. There was a yearning. The blank faces, I understood, but the yearning surprised me, and it hung in the air. Up until then, I had not allowed myself to dwell in this kind of space with nurses. My time with nurses had always been strategic around problems and solutions. I assumed that the problem solver me was what nurses wanted to see and hear. Instead I could feel an energy tug from the nurses. They wanted to talk more about meaning in their work. I wanted more of this space.

From there, this little question gave me a way into meaningful conversations about caring with nurses. I used it to open conversations when rounding and in nursing forums. To my surprise, nurses responded thoughtfully and with ease—even when on the fly. Some followed up with me when they had more time to answer and to tell a story about their authentic connections. My role as a leader of caring consciousness started to open up.

## Nursing Forums

I held nursing forums consistently as a CNO. They were scheduled every other month, on even months, on the third Thursday, twice during the afternoon, and twice during that night (Friday morning), at two o'clock and two forty-five. This way the staffs could switch out and cover for each other. Additional forums were scheduled during an odd month as needed. I opened each forum by handing out a *CNO Newsletter* that reported on hospital and nursing events, quality dashboards and projects, staff introductions, etc. These served as an agenda to get things started. Nurse attendance varied according to patient volumes and flow throughout the hospital. The night shifts were often more attended and more lively. This was an opportunity for everyone to speak. If one person dominated, I would move it along by going around the room for added comments. I always had flip chart paper on the walls where I wrote the nurses' thoughts, concerns, complaints, and suggestions as they stated them. I had learned that writing things on the flip chart papers where everyone can see helps to clarify the message or point, to keep conversations moving, to show people that they have been heard, and provide a clear list of follow-ups staff can expect. After the forums, the notes were typed up from the flip chart papers and sent to the nurse leaders and department heads to share and for needed follow-ups.

My authenticity and ease grew over time in the forums. In my early years in nursing administration, standing up in front of groups of outspoken nurses was scary. By the time I was a CNO, I was comfortable. I had the benefit of experience and the realization that the only barrier to authentic connection with nurses was me. I eventually realized several things about nurses and myself when holding open forums:

1. Nurses are fierce about issues they care about, rarely angry.
2. The more often I had the forums, the less tension there was.
3. I didn't need to know all the answers, and I didn't need to be right all the time.
4. I learned when to stop debating and to respond from within—what I valued, what I thought was right, and what I felt.
5. At one point, I knew that the quicker I dropped sounding like the company line, the quicker we connected to accomplish the change or goal at hand.
6. These forums were a time to be authentic with staff. Sometimes conversations were raw and contentious, which allowed honesty to surface.
7. This approach allowed the hard issues to be covered and all sides to be heard.

Nursing forums became a growing ground for my conscious caring role as a leader. I started to see myself differently and to trust the new direction. This put me in step with my original leadership purpose of helping nurses cultivate their caring practices.

## Rounding

Rounding was another avenue to connect meaningfully with nurses. For years I bounced around using different rounding approaches based on recent studies, books, or coaching advice in leadership journals. The challenge for me was to find meaningful topics that one could focus on with authenticity in short exchanges. We know that nurses see right through us when we try to connect with them inauthentically. Nurses know when we are collecting data versus being genuinely interested in them as people and nurses. Over the years, my rounding agendas had morphed from specific clinical indicators on a checklist to their professional goals, self-care practices, family events, and community interests. Those exchanges were good and sometimes meaningful but could land stale with no forward motion.

## Talking about Authentic Caring

An epiphany surfaced during a DAISY Award committee meeting. As we were reviewing authentic caring stories about our nurses, I realized that I would love to hear nurses talk about their caring stories. I thought if authentic caring is the goal, we could be talking with nurses about their caring experiences every day in real time. DAISY Awards[14] have significantly raised awareness of nurses' deep impact on patients and families through its formal recognition program. This recognition is important; however, it cannot fill the gap in voice and visibility of nurses' authentic caring throughout the industry.

Soon after, I started asking nurses about their caring experiences, one conversational experiment at a time. And to my delight, these questions shifted my connections with nurses. They palpably tapped into nurses' personal caring thoughts and feelings and touched on what motivated them and what was meaningful. This gave me a way into meaningful exchanges with nurses. These brief exchanges became a part of my rounding and nursing forums.

Authenticity and real connections are contagious when they are shared, and that contagion is within our reach. Authentic caring happens every day but not at the frequency or systemic level it could if it was a visible and talked about part of our work environments. All nurses, physicians and administrators would benefit from being a part of the stories in real time. DAISY Awards are important, but there's more.

## My Director's Team

Another positive in my CNO years was my nursing/clinical director leadership team; they reached high performance levels. They raised their team performance to the level of the strongest link, despite each being at different levels of leadership development. As a team they held themselves there through challenging times. They openly shared their resources and areas of expertise to the point of crescendo outcomes. I witnessed trust and generosity daily among them in staffing, patient flow decisions, and resource sharing. In crises, they banded together and stood like a pillar.

One event I especially enjoyed with them was holding nursing leadership retreats every six to nine months off site—usually in my home, attended by the directors of nursing, education, and quality. This was an opportunity to highlight the contextual forces that were driving the daily pressures that consumed us. In short order, I took time to paint a backdrop that connected the rise in science and technology, health care economics and reform, patient satisfaction, the emergence of wellness consciousness, and how nursing's social contract with society fit in. We reviewed principles, tools, and research from Watson's caring theory, caring science, *Quantum Leadership* by Porter-O'Grady and Malloch, and leadership materials from *The Advisory Board*. We sat in a circle each time reviewing the prepared handouts and sharing thoughts and feelings as I drew on flip chart paper posted on surrounding walls (as always).

I was convinced that if leaders could see their jobs within these contextual forces, it would help give their daily challenges a broader perspective and more meaning. One nursing director said, "I could sit here and listen and think about all of this all day long." Even though there was never enough time, these bits of consciousness cultivation impacted how we worked together. Because of our team connection, we were on track to take the organization forward. They were primed and ready to go. On the other hand, I suspected that this was not going to happen in this organization. The corporate walls were closing in on me.

# Chapter 13

# Alignments and Misalignments

Being a part of a health care corporation and networking with the other CNOs in the organization amplified my understanding of the national trends we were experiencing. Interest in how nurses delivered care was rising among our corporate leaders, not based on what we CNOs already knew or said but because of the monetization of patient satisfaction scores. It became clear that leaders in the health care industry at large were monitoring the rising data that reflected nurses' impact on patients. Suddenly nurses' caring practices were a commodity, and the health care industry leaders were paying attention.

## Nails on a Chalkboard

A crystallizing moment for me regarding patient satisfaction occurred at one of our organization's CNO quality leadership meetings in 2014. The CNO from Press Ganey[15] presented their recent nationwide patient satisfaction and experience data that illustrated cutting-edge trends and implications. Alas, it was confirmed that it was nurses' domain scores that drove overall patient scores in organizations. She explained that if the services delivered by nurses received high scores, the overall hospital scores were sure to be high. I sat there riveted. I wondered if the public's growing wellness consciousness and desire for authenticity in their care was playing out in these scores. Patients were telling us that their health care encounters were no longer all things medical. It was the nursing scores that carried the most weight, which provided public validation of nursing's value and impact on patients. The public was telling us that they were turning to nurses for authenticity and meaningful connections. Nursing's story was emerging in the patient satisfaction and experience data. What initially felt like a revelation to me suddenly echoed, *Wait, I know what this is; this is caring science in action.*

When I returned home from the conference, I started poring through nursing leadership journals about caring with new eyes. I wanted to find leadership journal articles championing this monumental pivot point for nursing in the industry. I was looking for a new direction. But it was in this context that finding repeated articles promoting scripted, formulaic caring programs in leadership journals that felt like nails on a chalkboard. The programs in the articles were designed to increase patient satisfaction scores, not to reach higher levels of caring, not to respond to patients' need for authenticity or to tap into nursing's essence. They were not based on caring science. I was disappointed.

My CNO experiences illustrated that nurses are motivated to provide high-quality caring, but they need avenues to learn how to balance the demands of their work.

It's not their organizations' mission statements that motivate them; it's their individual caring experiences with patients that cultivate a yearning to expand their caring practices. Nurse leaders' first consideration should be nurses' existing caring skills and motivation. This provides an authentic basis on which to build caring initiatives.

## Time to Resign

As for my job, resigning from my CNO position had become my only option in 2015. After the union assessment had come and gone, the target on my back could not be erased. There are many layers in leadership roles. Not all the layers have to be aligned to lead authentically. But for a CNO, there is one thing that must be aligned, and that is organizational fit. I was not a fit with these corporate leaders and the CEO.

# CHAPTER 14

# I Finally Jumped!

When I ask myself, where was my mind all those years? My answer flashes to the boiling frog parable. The myth is that if a frog is put into a pan of tepid water while coming to a boil, the frog's body adjusts to the rising temperature and the frog will remain in the simmering water and die. However, if the frog is lowered into boiling water, it will immediately jump out of the water to save itself. I lived a life in the simmering water of the health care industry for years. I believe many nurse leaders live this same life. I didn't have the sense to jump out of the boiling water, until I did.

## My Call to Action

For too long, the rising heat generated by the pace and intensity of the health care industry had distracted me from finding ways to apply caring science in my leadership. I had to find incremental ways to lead authentic caring. It started in my CNO position. One advantage to being a CNO is that it's only you at the top, so you have to trust yourself. It was in this role that I said to myself, "If I deeply believe in the importance of authentic caring for patients and nurses, I must act. Even though we are mired in conflicting demands, I can at least talk more about authentic caring. And even though I may not know how as a CNO to help nurses expand their authentic caring skills, I can explore it." Once I realized that if I didn't start engaging in caring as a leader, then who would? This is when I jumped.

## Four Obstacles Turned to Lessons

To get on the road less traveled of authentic caring leadership, I had to work through several belief systems that had become obstacles. These turned into lessons learned. The first lesson was that my job demands and heavy workloads were not what were holding me back from leading caring. It was more about allowing myself to think and talk about authentic caring and threading it through everyday conversations and decisions. I started with my nurse leadership team, in our meetings. Then I integrated questions and conversations about authentic caring into classes I taught, then into nursing forums, during rounding, with my executive peers and occasionally in board meetings. Leading caring in increments shifted my mind-set, which shifted my perceptions of my job demands and workloads. Connecting with nurses in meaningful ways motivated me to connect more, to round more, to talk more with nurses about caring, and to think more about caring.

The second obstacle I had to grapple with was thinking nurses didn't have time for more authentic caring moments. This is a tough bias to unwind. Authentic caring is about brief moments that can have lasting effects. It's making connections in between nursing's active work. It's more about incremental awareness than it is about time. That's why each nurse has to discover this individually. Leaders being there to lend credibility and affirmation to the incremental discoveries by nurses can make the difference. As nurses expand their awareness and ability to authentically engage with patients around the demands of their work, we can be more accessible to say, "Wow."

The third obstacle was the fear that I did not have the capacity or skills to help others achieve authentic caring. The only way through this fear was to trust the process. Once I started talking, asking, and sharing thoughts and observations about authentic caring, I saw caring energy spark in other nurses and leaders, and I was launched. From there I learned how to explore with nurses how they achieved their authenticity and caring connections. These short, meaningful conversations with nurses showed me the way to impact others' authenticity and connections. As we make known what caring is and its dynamics in our own lives, this ripples through others. Everyone's capacity for authenticity and authentic caring connection strengthens, especially our own.

The fourth obstacle that had held me back was the reality that cultivation of the capacity for authentic caring is each nurse's personal responsibility. This reality prevented me from seeing the nurse leaders' role in nurses' personal journeys. An authentic, caring work environment is a two-part dance. Nurse leaders' role is to create an environment where there is visibility around authentic caring. Giving voice to authentic caring in daily conversations from classrooms to the bedside and to boardrooms attracts nurses and others. Asking questions, sharing stories, and prompting descriptions of the mechanics and magic of authentically connecting with patients carries meaning to others. And although nurses' cultivation of their authentic caring skills is personal, individual, and voluntary, leaders' conversations spark curiosity and adoption of caring thoughts and actions for many nurses. These four obstacles kept me in the boiling water and prevented me from focusing more on the right things. As these beliefs dissipated, I was freed to see more possibilities for caring.

## My Leadership Journey Landed

Who we are is how we lead. And there you have it. This was my reality and is at the core of my story. My leader self couldn't escape me. This reality is the first of seven core realities in the framework of complexity leadership described by Crowell.[16] This framework provided missing pieces in my leadership puzzle. I had studied complexity science in school and had reveled in this context when learning the nature of nursing— its dynamic systems, patterns and relationships, spontaneous activities, nonlinear behaviors, and more. Understanding nursing and nurse leadership in this context helped me make sense of my career.

Learning the wisdom behind the futility of trying to control chaos and change was another complexity leadership reality I was exposed to. Controlling, adapting, and surviving in health care had been my career's mantra. I even found "helping nurses adapt in health care's chaos" as one of my written goals in a 1999 Franklin Planner. I had to learn this lesson the hard way. Trying to control put me on a slippery slope, one of losing sight of the essence of nursing. Even though I studied caring science, the leadership signals in nursing journals and books focused on structure and perceived control. I needed to feel in control, like the other nurse leaders in the journals.

But not Alice Davidson. She tried to help me release the controls that held me back from caring science engagement. Alice was my teacher/mentor in my last two DNP courses at CU. She was a quantum mechanics scholar and helped me develop a complexity science leadership model customized for my work setting. Alice was creator and an editor of the 2011 book, *Nursing, Caring, and Complexity Science* (Davidson, Ray, and Turkel).[17] She died before the book was published. She had written me a note after I graduated in 2006 about how she and a peer were working on a book and that it would have authors like Liehr and Smith, whom we had studied in class. Did she know I would benefit from this book? Here I am ten years later, reading complexity leadership and story theory by Liehr and Smith[18] in Alice's book, and learning how to tell my story. I believe Alice is still urging me on. Thank you, Alice.

I hope that by telling my story, readers—nurse leaders and nurses—will consider their own stories. Maybe new paths to deeper authenticity and renewed connections among nurse leaders and nurses in organizations will reveal themselves. Authentic caring and relationships can be found and resurrected in any group of nurses. It's there.

## Who Am I 2.0?

Taking responsibility for one's thoughts and actions is a universal pivot point in any person's life toward health, life balance, and wellness. I started turning this corner slowly in my personal life using self-help books and then more advanced self-care therapies and practices along the way. I'm still on the path of more self-acceptance and being comfortable in vulnerability so I can go deeper into authenticity and connection with others. I hope to meet myself at some point as I turn more corners in self-growth. My wellness and healing efforts have had the most benefit and meaning to me with my daughters. They are both thriving in their lives. Our older daughter is a yoga practitioner, energy worker, and painter. Our younger daughter is a nursing PhD student with a focus on reproductive rights and global health. As parents of these two smart, strong-minded women in our complicated world of male domination and patriarchy, it's satisfying to watch them take the baton. David and I are still rising to be our best. We've been at this for forty-five years and plan to continue. Truth be told, David often muses that the reason we made it this far together is because he was away much of the time. Who knows? We're going strong now, working on our individual missions and projects, and "living the dream"—another David saying.

# PART V

## THE BIGGER STORY— OUR FUTURE

# CHAPTER 15

# Into the Future

As health care chaos and reform were coming to a head, the Robert Wood Johnson Foundation [19] and the Institute of Medicine [20] were working on "The Future of Nursing: Leading Change, Advancing Health," published in 2010.[21] Their purpose was to assess and transform nursing in ways that would allow expansion of quality health care to all Americans. The aim was to "usher in the golden age of nursing," to position nurses not only as trusted professionals at the bedside but as front-line activists, change agents, and leaders in the health care reform movement (Johnson et al., 2012).[22] The report encompassed four areas: expansion of nursing practice and roles, higher nurse education levels, more participation in leadership partnerships, and effective workforce planning and policy based on better information infrastructures. Not surprisingly, there has been pushback over the last eight years from medicine, health care organizations, and others. It's understandable; the IOM proclamations to raise nursing standards in practice, education, and leadership come at a time when patient demographics are mushrooming, baby boom nurses are retiring, health care reform obstacles are around every corner, and social political uncertainty is looming. The stakes are high for people's health and for nursing. But if we don't act now, then when?

## RNs Needed

There are now 3.1 million working registered nurses (RNs) in the United States with a projected need for 712,000 more to fill new jobs associated with demographic changes and health care growth. And another 495,000 RNs are needed by 2020 to replace the anticipated RN retirees according to *The State of Nursing 2016—White Paper* by Nursing.org.[23] Raising retention to the top of the to-do list could not be more critical.

## What Drives Us Out of Nursing

The IOM authors acknowledged the importance of nurse retention to achieve their new standards in nursing practice, education, leadership, and infrastructure. They spoke to the destabilizing impact of nurse turnover on nurses, patient quality, and health care costs, and questioned why retention programs were not more widely implemented. Their report illustrated that 40 percent of nurses leave nursing because of workplace conditions, and the remaining reasons were for personal career decisions or family needs.[21] The IOM spoke to the environmental variables that dominate nurse turnover and attrition research, the things that drive us out of nursing—staffing, schedules, workloads, inefficiencies, technology, communications, disruptive behaviors, etc. For solutions, the IOM turned to the strategies known in nursing organizations and research for advancing structural empowerment, nursing professional and leadership development, and improving work environments—shared governance, Magnet recognition, Transforming Care at the Bedside, and the Center for Nursing Excellence, among others.[24] These programs have had a profound impact in raising nursing's professional standards and mitigating environmental obstacles and stressors. They have generated over two decades of research on the triple wins of reducing nurse turnover, improving patient outcomes, and lowering costs. But something is missing.

These structural programs have not uniformly addressed the intrinsic nature and behavioral dynamics of nurses' caring. Traditional strategies have been more about nurses surviving the external elements that affect them within the health care industry—work environments and professional development—than about their internal and interpersonal resources. This is problematic as avoiding the cultivation of nurses' inner resources creates a gap in our professional narrative of how to thrive in nursing. The Advisory Board Company [25] touched on this nurse engagement gap. They identified that stress reduction and burnout were the areas of lowest success in nurse engagement across 575 health care organizations (Koppel et al. 2015, 534).[26] Retention depends on the engagement of nurses. Nurse engagement is generated from two primary sources: organizational resources that mitigate job stressors and support professional growth and autonomy, and nurses' inner resources that support personal growth and self-worth (AACN, UWES).[27,28] It is the second requirement of engagement that nursing leadership in the industry at large has not addressed. There's no doubt that nurses' internal mechanisms of stress and stress relief are complex and are interactive and reactive to job stressors. We as leaders not only have to mitigate the job stressors that drive nurses out of nursing; we must also learn how to cultivate what keeps nurses in nursing.

# CHAPTER 16

# What Keeps Us In Nursing

Nursing attracts nurses for a lot of different reasons. There are the bells and whistles, saving lives and quality of life, the science and research, the salaries, job flexibility, and job security. But above all of these is the desire to tap into something greater than themselves. This is the desire that carries the most weight, and yet we continue to get it so wrong.

Daniel Pink, in his book *Drive: The Surprising Truth About What Motivates Us* describes how wrong we are in the way we are leading our twenty-first-century individuals across all industries (2009).[29] He says that there is a vast disconnect between motivation science and what businesses do. It is the intrinsic drivers—the internal, organic, and essential—that motivate our younger generations to stay. (And I contend, all generations.) Is there another profession more intrinsically motivated than nursing? This is a time to acknowledge what keeps us in nursing and build our retention strategies around those desires and forces.

## For the Joy of It

The hard realities of burnout and attrition hit home at the Institute for Healthcare Improvement (IHI) in 2014.[30] They progressed their Triple Aim initiatives to the Quadruple Aim to address the high rates of nurse and physician burnout and attrition that are threatening health care outcomes. Reports showed a range of 30 to 50 percent of new nurses and 54 to 60 percent of physicians were thinking of leaving their jobs or professions (Brown et al., 2018; Kabcenell, Perlo, and Sakallaris, 2016).[31, 2] The IHI understood that their Triple Aim initiatives—the patient experience, patient health, and cost reduction—were being impacted by the personal states of the caregivers. This led them to their fourth aim, caregivers' health, how caregivers care for themselves. Their diagnosis: burnout has reached epidemic levels, turnover is up, and morale is down (Perlo et al., 2017,5).[32] From there, what was really refreshing was the strategy they chose, one designed to reengage caregivers' intrinsic motivators in their work. They chose joy. This is right in line with Pink's intrinsic motivation science, "for the joy of it." The IHI's goal is to leverage joy—an asset they describe as living within the caregiver—to help access meaning and purpose in patient care. And their strategy to help caregivers find joy is through conversation. On top of their trademark tools and improvement practices, they added having conversations with caregivers about what matters most to them and how they find meaning and purpose in their work. This is the right direction.

## The Sweet Spot Where Nurses Thrive

For nurses, our path to joy is most alive in our authentic caring practices. Nurses find science interesting and challenging, but it's the human connections and caring that bring the sense of purpose and meaning to nurses (Galuska et al., 2018,157).[33] The meaning and impact of the caring connections involved in the nurse-patient relationship were defined and validated in the pioneering study by Halldorsdottir (1991, 39).[34] It provided a language for the levels and the dynamics of patients' and nurses' shared experiences in the caring process. These details help us understand the complexity of the experiences and make them real and visible. The study defined five levels ranging from uncaring to caring (biocidic, biostatic, biopassive, bioactive, and biogenic). The biocidic level (life-destroying) is where the nurse causes distress for the patient. The biostatic mode (life-restraining) is created by an insensitive or indifferent nurse. The biopassive level (life neutral) reflects "It's just a job" behaviors. The bioactive level (life-sustaining) of caring is given by a nurse who is kind, concerned, reassuring, and responsive to patients' needs. These are the type of desired nurse characteristics defined in scripted formulaic caring programs used in health care organizations to standardize caring and to maximize patient satisfaction scores. And the highest level of the caring relationships is biogenic. This level of caring is consistent with what experts describe in authentic caring moments and the transpersonal caring relationship (Watson 2012).[35] What sets biogenic caring apart from all other levels of caring is its life-giving and life-receiving nature for both the nurse and patient. Authentic caring connections originate within the nurse, spark from a connection between the nurse and patient, are cultivated through the nurses' inner resources and caring consciousness, and can recommit nurses to nursing in the process. Many of us know the power of such a mechanism—one that nurtures nurses' caring capacity through authentic connections; is directly aligned with our patients' expanding caring needs and expectations; and has the ability to motivate nurses to remain in nursing by intrinsically rewarding them through their work in real time.

Nurses experiencing a sense of well-being related to having a meaningful impact on a patient or situation is not uncommon (Amendolair 2012),[36] even to the point of sustaining their desire to stay in nursing (Dotson et al. 2014).[37] Twenty-seven nurses provided stories through StoryCorps that reflected the same connection between their sense of meaning and joy when their care benefited their patients (Galuska et al. 2018).[33] These reciprocal connections between nurse and other through authentic caring are what restore trust, faith, and hope (Watson, 2012).[35]

## Nurses' Journey to Authentic Caring

The journey to authentic caring is individual and personal. It starts with the nurse's initial desire to help people. In school, authentic caring is introduced and cultivated through acquiring knowledge, experiences with patients, and reflection. But once employed in health care, support of authentic caring cultivation too often suspends. From there, it can be a lonely journey for nurses to cultivate their inner resources and sustain their authentic caring. Authentic caring certainly exists today but not at the frequency or systemic level it could if it was a conscious and visible part of our work environments.

It is true that nurses' desire to authentically care is often greater than their inner resources. This creates confusion, frustration, and a sense of lack of control that can lead nurses to blame their jobs and organizations, their leaders, their peers, and at its worst, their patients. These reactions contribute to nurse burnout, compassion fatigue, moral distress (Kester and Wei 2018),[38] and even depression. Nurses' depression rates are double that of the general public (Magtibay et al. 2017).[39] These emotional states hold nurses back from their authenticity and diminish their ability to connect with patients and others, impacting patient care, and putting them at risk to leave nursing. Burnout doesn't happen because we care too much; it happens because we wall ourselves off from human connectedness, where our inner resources are replenished and cultivated (Watson 2016).[40] This is not just about job satisfaction; it is about nurses learning how to thrive in nursing. It involves caring consciousness cultivation through self-care and support from within the work environment and nursing community.

# CHAPTER 17

# Self-Care Is Required for Self and Caring

Cultivation of nurses' inner resources and caring consciousness starts with self-care. It is well established in nursing and self-care literature that how nurses relate to themselves impacts their quality of connections and relationships and the care they provide. Personal knowledge is required for authentic caring and is facilitated through self-care and in relationships with others. "One can only understand in another what is understood in self" (Eckroth-Bucher 2010, 297).[41] Our current lifestyles certainly reinforce this correlation. Wellness programs and lifestyle research abound that demonstrate connections between personal growth, self-care practices, self-acceptance, quality of relationships, and quality of life. This explains the personal renaissance happening around us evident in the groundswell of wellness programs in our society in all walks of life. There is no way around it: authentic caring starts with self, and lifelong self-care is the prescription for growing.

Self-care practices are multifaceted and highly individual—each practice affects each person uniquely—and range across a continuum. Self-care involves physical, mind/mental/emotional, and spiritual care practices. Basically self-care can be what individuals define as something they do for themselves to be healthier. To understand self-care practices, it's helpful to see them by categories based on desired intention and purpose. One does not need to approach self-care practices linearly by category; in fact, they are often in motion simultaneously and can be synergistic. Here are general categories of self-care practices:

- Self-care for prevention: The intention of all self-care practices is to prevent and reduce the accumulation of stress hormones in our bodies related to threat (vulnerability) and stress. Chronic stress has debilitating effects on our health. Practices in any of the physical, emotional, or spiritual realms affect the whole. Practices may include: balanced nutrition, physical exercise, stress management, self-compassion, mindfulness, meditation, reflection, yoga, massage, bio-energy practices (Reiki, healing touch), time in nature, the arts (music, literature, writing, theatre, fine arts), creative aesthetic endeavors, spiritual practices, and social, religious, community engagement, and beyond.

- Therapeutic self-care for life struggles: The goal of these self-care practices is to address barriers, vulnerabilities, conflicts, disruptions in daily life around relationships, changes or decisions that may require therapy, counseling, or programs for behavior change. Therapy and counseling are strengthened by concurrent use of other self-care practices that support physical, emotional, and spiritual health as listed above.

- Developmental self-care to advance life skills: These are practices designed to enhance balance and satisfaction in our lives and in our work through self-development and growth. These skills help convert hollow practices and resistance into productive inner-growth experiences. Self-development skills are facilitated by emotional intelligence programs, mind-body science, and self-help, and are supported by other self-care practices.

- Transformative self-care toward wholeness: This path of lifelong learning is one of transcendent growth toward achievement of our fullest potential of positive emotions, fulfillment, meaning, love of humanity, relationships, and spirituality. Well-being is the state of integration and balance within mind, body, and spirit. Common practices include mindfulness and meditation and are supported by all other self-care. One arrives at wholeness through wellness, healing, and well-being.

Self-care practices have long been associated with cultivating nurses' inner resources, reducing stress, and enhancing authentic caring. Nurses who achieved health-promotion behaviors and perspectives through self-care practices showed lower levels of compassion fatigue, burnout, and stress, and higher compassion satisfaction and job satisfaction in three health promotion behaviors model (HPB) studies. The self-care domains were nutrition, stress management, spiritual growth (achieving meaning, purpose, and life goals), health responsibility, physical activity, and interpersonal relations. The deeper intrinsic HPB domains of spiritual growth and interpersonal relationships had the greatest impact on nurses and led to a sense of intimacy, closeness, and meaningful relationships that align with authentic connections and caring (Tucker et al., 2012; Neville and Cole 2013; Williams et al., 2018).[42,43,44] Resilience in clinical practice is often a byproduct of nurses' self-care practices, such as education, social support, self-care activities, fostering relationships, boundary setting, resilience training, learning stress control, and engaging in debriefs (Kester and Wei 2018).[38] Whether these self-care techniques are offered through an employer or outside, they are practices that can help nurses and leaders navigate work demands and wholly engage in their work.

Nurse leader burnout is a growing concern. Nurse leaders are critical given the IOM's call for stronger nurse leadership in health care in number and position. It is estimated that we need 67,000 additional nurse managers by 2020 (Nursing.org).[23] This poses a challenge given nurse manager turnover is between 50 to 72 percent (McCright, Pabico, and Roux, 2018; Warshawsky and Havens, 2014).[45,4] Articles advising nurse leaders to seek joy through use of self-care, resilience, and self-management to avoid burnout have multiplied since the IHI Quadruple Aim came out, each with a different twist. A caring philosophy—based in caring science—was attributed to twenty CNOs' high-level resilience and leadership success. "A lifelong process of fine-tuning the art of caring in nursing leadership" was their mantra (Dyess et al., 2015, 106).[46] These studies illustrate that nurse leaders benefit from the same use of self-care, resilience practices, and caring science processes as clinical nurses. Cultivation of inner resources is a universal need.

# CHAPTER 18

# Our Twenty-First-Century Legacy—Nurses Thriving

Nursing is ever evolving. Nursing parallels the evolution of the human experience and society's health, healing, and caring needs within the consciousness of the time. Through history, nursing has designed and provided caregiving individually and collectively for those affected by illness, injury, disability, and beyond. Nursing involves the balance of each person's personal, physical, and environmental capabilities and resources, while ensuring safety, autonomy, and sustaining the whole person. In each phase of history, the essence of nursing has been authentic caring, making real connections with patients. Over recent decades, however, the rapid rise of science and technology and the stronghold of business demands have restrained nursing's collective voice around authentic caring within the health care industry. The tides are now turning.

We are experiencing a cultural wellness renaissance in our society evident in the groundswell of wellness programs in all walks of life. Patients are recognizing that health isn't just absence of disease and illness; it is integrative health, mind-body-spirit health. Patients want more than medical care in their health care encounters; they are seeking holistic responses, and they are turning to nurses for that sense of well-being and wholeness amid the turmoil. These moments align with nursing's essence: authentic caring. Jean Watson said decades ago, "The change will come when nursing and nurses are directly aligned with the people they serve" (1999, 46).[1]

Understanding these contextual forces brings nurse leaders to a new territory, one of legacy, a legacy of nurses thriving in nursing. Do we not have an obligation to make standard that which we know will help nurses thrive in nursing? We know that the health care industry is a beast to work in, that real, caring experiences are far too few, and that authentic caring connections create a sense of well-being for both patient and nurse. What we have not recognized is the strong influence nurse leaders within health care organizations can have in creating environments where authentic caring can thrive. Academicians and educators have been sounding the benefits of caring science, research, and processes to nurses and students for decades. But the seas are too rough and the noise is too loud amid the work demands for nurse leaders to hear the call. But we must. If we nurse leaders want nurses to focus on authentic caring, then we must focus on it as leaders. Nurse leaders giving voice to authentic caring with their unique influence and credibility in nurses' work environments can capture nurses' attention and imagination and serve a role in reconnecting nurses to their purpose. Nurse leaders are in the best position to make authentic caring's invisibility visible and the unrealistic real in health care. Nurse leaders can ebb the tide of attrition.

Retention is our top priority for nurses, patients, health care, and society, despite all other worthy priorities nurse leaders are consumed in. If attrition trends are not reversed, the other priorities won't matter. We cannot sidestep this looming obligation. Retention in the twenty-first century calls nurse leaders to engage in nurses' caring consciousness cultivation. Our role is to tap into nurses' deep motivations and open paths for nurses to cultivate their inner resources so they can access their purpose and authenticity—even when stressed—and learn to thrive in nursing. This is our twenty-first-century legacy. We can turn the tide of authentic caring in health care and save nurses from leaving nursing.

## PART VI

# A NURSE LEADER LEGACY

## CHAPTER 19

# A Call to Action

This book is based on my experiences as a nurse leader and student of caring science through the steep growth trajectory of science and technology in the health care industry. It responds to the vacuum of an authentic caring focus within the health care industry. It comes with a sense of urgency and need to make the leadership of authentic caring realistic and doable for nurse leaders, and real for nurses. The pace and complexity in nurses' jobs leave too many nurses feeling disconnected from their original purpose in being a nurse, and searching for ways to leave nursing. At the same time, wellness forces in our society are shifting health care and aligning patients to seek and recognize nurses' authentic caring—aligning nurses more closely with the people we serve. This is a call for nurse leaders to fill this gap that leads nurses to search elsewhere for purpose and meaning. This is a call to action for the benefit of nurses, patients, and society.

## Leading Authentic Caring Today

How we mainstream caring consciousness cultivation in today's nursing work environments and cultures has been a lingering question within nursing throughout my career. The prevailing answer has been to leave it to each nurse as his/her responsibility—given that caring cultivation is personal and voluntary. This singular approach is no longer an option. Nurses need help in navigating caring consciousness endeavors within our high-paced technical work environments. The time is now, and nurse leaders are in the best position to help them.

What holds us back? The summary version is that nurse leaders within the health care industry are caught in a revolving quagmire of four competing mind-sets in how to cultivate caring. First, organizations primarily support and fund caring initiatives that are concrete and can be managed in traditional ways. Second, nurses believe that it is the job demands that prevent them from connecting authentically with patients more often. Third, nursing education systems promote the use of caring science and its principles in nursing organizations' professional practice and caring programs, but implementation rarely gets beyond the planning and approval stages. And fourth, nurse leaders within the health care industry work hard to conform to recommendations from outside standard setting organizations, but underneath it all, many nurse leaders do not see caring science and nursing theories as realistic paths to lead nurse caring in their organizations. As a result, there are few paths for caring cultivation in health care industry settings.

However, there are exceptions. Several hospitals across the country have aligned with organizations that provide programs that cultivate higher levels of caring, healing, and holistic and integrative care. The two organizations most recognized for providing integrated programs in health care systems are from the Watson Caring Science Institute (WCSI)[47] and the American Holistic Nurse Association (AHNA).[48] They have similar missions: to expand and improve caring throughout health care locally and internationally. The WCSI is a membership organization that has over 150 health care facilities engaged at the affiliate and associate levels; has partnerships with education systems and organizations; has certified over 430 Caritas Coaches through the Caritas Coaching Education Program (CCEP),[49] and holds an annual educational conference. The WCSI was founded by Jean Watson and supports a growing body of human caring theory, caring science, and Caritas publications, programs, and scholars. The AHNA is also a membership organization that has provided over 1,050 certifications for a number of levels of holistic nurse practices. They provide endorsements for schools, issue an annual award for institutional excellence to qualifying health care organizations, and hold an annual educational conference. These organizations have had a significant impact on nursing and our health care system by generating recognition, research, literature, standards, and quality for holistic caring and healing. In addition to these comprehensive programs, there are consulting companies and individuals that offer staff and system development services designed to improve care in health care organizations.

## The Scope of This Challenge

Despite this progress, the scope of this challenge remains immense. To put it in perspective, nationwide there are 6,210 hospitals, 410,000 nurse leaders, and 3.1 million nurses—with evidence suggesting that nearly half of these are wishing to leave nursing.[31] This calls for not just one additional approach to help nurses learn to thrive in nursing, but for many new approaches.

There is a lot of territory to cover. Ideally, the goal is to help all nurses thrive in nursing, and we can start with one nurse at a time within each organization. Expanding access to caring consciousness cultivation for nurses beyond our current reach is the mission. Nurses thriving in nursing starts with helping them cultivate their caring consciousness at the grassroots level to enrich the meaning and purpose in their work. The steps can be organic, locally grown and weave collateral pathways that connect more nurse leaders and more nurses to the mission.

## One Step Forward

The human mind tends to gravitate to the complex, and yet it is in the basics where transformation occurs. My goal here is to make available some of the basics that I have learned from my nurse leadership experiences and from caring science. I have benefitted from studying caring science in my doctorate education and more recently by completing the CCEP.[49] But not all nurse leaders are surrounded with caring science resources or believe in the various theories and philosophies related to caring science. I suspect that I made caring science more complex than need be, which kept me from accessing it in my leadership for many years. My story shows that having access to those resources does not automatically produce a leader of caring. Through my experiences, I see that caring science is the study of what lives within each nurse and nurse leader. I believe that each nurse leader can build on the caring capacity nurses bring to nursing and help nurses grow their inner resources and caring consciousness. I know from experience that an authentic connection between a nurse leader and nurse can put a nurse on a path of learning how to thrive in nursing.

Here is one plan; it represents one-step forward in our health care landscape, a landscape with a lot of ground to cover. This plan is simple and is based on authentic caring basics. It focuses on tapping into nurses' existing caring motivation to connect with others; it is doable for leaders and is real for nurses. Nurse leaders in any setting can use it. It's the practice of caring engagement conversations. These conversations can take nurse leaders and nurses forward one step at a time. It is a grassroots, organic, nurse-led practice that starts with nurse leaders where they are comfortable in their caring consciousness. It rises from within each leader and can be used in conjunction with other caring initiatives or as a stand-alone practice. This one-step forward provides a path for nurse leaders to help themselves and nurses to slow things down and have short routine conversations about what matters most about being a nurse—caring. There is nothing new in this nurse leader practice; it threads through nursing's history since Nightingale and is relevant today. It can help us help nurses thrive in nursing in today's work environments.

Conversations about caring between nurse leaders and nurses have always been important but have been squeezed out by other demands. Our work settings have become void of the language of caring—authenticity, voicing feelings, identifying vulnerabilities, seeking meaning. Nurse leaders can take the lead and help themselves and nurses by using caring engagement conversations. This proved true in one critical care department where caring culture gaps were identified in their work setting. Knowing that nurses and nurse leaders were often distracted from what matters most, the nurse leaders used caring engagement conversations as a solution. "Allowing nurses to recognize the duality of the nurse-patient relationship, the giving and taking from one another, is an important element of healing and growth" (Mason et al 2014, 223).[50] Over time their measurement of caring fatigue among the nurses in the department improved. The goal and success of these conversations went beneath the surface and tapped into the motivations that brought nurses into nursing in the first place.

When I was a CNO, there were several things that came together that prompted me to start giving voice to authentic caring on a routine basis and to start asking nurses about their authentic caring experiences, thoughts, and feelings. These were pivotal moments that triggered me to start leading caring in my own way. My realization was, if I believed in the reciprocal benefits of authentic caring for patients and nurses, then I needed to give voice to that and to engage nurses around it. My beginning steps were rudimentary, but it was enough to get me started. This was a way to grow authentic caring as a nurse leader. These caring engagement conversations showed me nurses' humanity and their hardships in a new light. I felt better about myself and about each nurse and all nurses. Nurses responded in surprising and refreshing ways that showed a desire for connection and authenticity. My world opened up.

My hope is that this book will inspire nurse leaders to give voice to authentic caring with nurses in their organizations and use it as an opportunity to expand caring consciousness within themselves and among their fellow nurses. I also hope that nurse leaders will find joy and meaning in their reflective conversations with nurses and make these exchanges a part of their legacy. "A legacy is not a big grand thing; it's in every life we touch" (Maya Angelou, Witherspoon 2014).[51]

## Develop a Network of Like-Minded Nurse Leaders

As a leader, all roads lead back to being open, honest, and authentic with ourselves, our leadership team, and nurses. Learning how to generate trusting work relationships has been part of my life's journey. Opening up with nurses about my inner thoughts and feelings about authentic caring was part of that journey.

Leading with a more visible demonstration of one's caring consciousness creates a strong gravitational pull. It attracts like-minded nurse leaders and nurses and some skeptics. Having a few simpatico leaders to fall back on for support when one is feeling vulnerable is required to keep oneself open and thriving as a leader. There are two questions to ask yourself when identifying authentic and healthy teammates: Who has your best interests in mind? Who will tell you the truth? Our goal as a nurse leader is to help nurses thrive in nursing. First we must demonstrate to nurses what thriving in relationships and nursing look like.

# CHAPTER 20

# The Basics of Caring Engagement Conversations

The basics to caring engagement conversations involve asking nurses to share their authentic caring experiences, thoughts, and feelings. Helping others name their thoughts, expectations, needs, and feelings without judgment provides clarification and is a critical component in discovery. The process of translating thoughts and feelings around an event with a simple, caring literacy word or label helps raise awareness, anchors and grows understanding and expands caring consciousness. The process of knowing that one is being heard is where healing occurs. I saw this as a nurse leader. Once nurses felt authentically heard with no judgment or correction, the possibilities of self-discovery opened up.

What makes this approach doable is that nurse leaders are already rounding and talking with nurses in various settings. By shifting conversations with nurses to caring engagement conversations nurses will respond differently. Caring and especially authentic caring has a universal draw among nurses. Nurses lean in even in momentary and episodic exchanges. These conversations can help set the stage for broader organizational integration of caring science programs if and when they occur. Regardless, the greater mission of helping nurses cultivate their purpose and meaning in nursing in any setting and scope moves nursing and nurses forward and helps us keep nurses in nursing.

## What It Is and Is Not

The focus of this leadership practice is nurse-centered. The nurse leader starts by tapping into nurses' existing beliefs, thoughts, feelings, and values that drive their caring practices. An environment of appreciation and awareness of the individual nurses' caring practices develops when we ask about and listen to their feelings, values, and perceptions. Words are clarified and built upon and emerge into a caring language.

Keeping the conversations nurse-centered does not diminish the importance of patient-centered care, it provides a balance. Our current emphasis on patient-centered care and other caring programs without equal time with nurses on their existing caring practices undermines respect for what nurses are already doing and creates a gap in trust between nurses and leaders. I found that nurses are hungry for opportunities to tell leaders how they care and to reflect on their process. Nurse leaders talking about and listening to what brings meaning to nurses, and giving time to authentically reflect on feelings and thoughts, creates relationships, expands perspectives, and deepens caring consciousness. Organizations are steeped in initiatives that tell nurses how they should care; this is not that.

## Who Better to Do the Engaging

Given the immediacy of the need and the resistant nature for change within the health care industry, nurse leaders from within the industry are in the best position to recalibrate caring cultivation amid the intense clinical demands. Nurse leaders have the influence and credibility to "give permission" to pause and access their original intentions and purpose through conversations. These are conversations that go beneath the surface and tap into the motivations that brought nurses into nursing in the first place. This is a different way to lead caring. Nurse leaders are invited to share their own purpose with nurses and for nurses to share theirs. Nurse leaders don't have to be gurus; they just need to be willing and authentic. Nurse leaders start where they are, and the comfort levels will grow. "Show your humanity and no one will turn away" (Doty, 2017).[52]

## The When and Where

Waiting for the best place and time to talk about authentic caring with nurses is a dilemma for most nurse leaders and educators. I propose to just jump in. These reflective conversations between nurse leaders and nurses are designed to be momentary and episodic, in-between patients and meetings. They happen in hallways when rounding, in classrooms when teaching, and in conference rooms when meeting. This is a big ask. Nurse leaders commonly believe that meaningful conversations with nurses cannot happen in these spaces and time. But they can. These short reflective conversations rise in the same way nurses connect with patients in authentic and meaningful ways. Just as authentic caring moments are doable between nurses and patients in busy clinical settings, so it goes between leaders and nurses.

## How to Start

Asking nurses about their authentic caring was a new approach for me. I was uncertain if nurses would be annoyed by such an inward, thoughtful question in the middle of their busy work demands. I hoped that navigating different consciousness levels would not be foreign to them. My hunch was right. The nurses leaned in.

The first step is for nurse leaders to engage nurses with questions that tap into nurses' existing caring practices, and then to listen and appreciate how nurses see and interpret their caring experiences. Sharing and translating nurses' caring experiences into caring literate words and concepts will emerge into caring language. These reflective conversations between nurses and leaders create a new narrative of mutual authenticity and caring consciousness and literacy in real time.

My process of initiating these conversations started with a question with nurses about their views and intentionality around their caring practices, followed by a pause. The microsecond pause let me know if the nurse could shift or needed to stay focused on the clinical. The nurses intuitively knew that this was not just face time, or the next flavor of the month. These became human exchanges, not boss–worker exchanges. Several nurses were immediately forthcoming with ease and efficiency. Others looked bewildered, as if they hadn't considered their thoughts about caring for some time. And others passed on the opportunity. Some nurses, who refrained initially, shared the next time I came around. The more often I asked about real caring, the more often nurses participated. There were awkward times. It was one experimental, casual conversation at a time. This showed me that even though nurses are busy, the nature of the topic drew many nurses in. I am convinced that there are nurses from all specialties who long to converse about their caring thoughts and experiences. It's our job to invite them to share.

Knowing how to invite nurses into casual, meaningful conversations about caring is leader specific. Every leader and every conversation will look different. Authentic caring is personal and requires some thought. This is not an initiative rollout; there are no endgames or measurements. The "script" lives in you. It comes from your caring consciousness and is the reason you are a nurse leader—to impact nurses' work and lives for the better. However, it is helpful to have your own thoughts and perspectives ready to propel others to talk if needed. These conversations are not an exercise in full disclosure of all your thoughts and feelings on caring. Less is more—another David saying.

The scope of this nurse leader practice can be a lone nurse having conversations with fellow nurses; it can be a unit or department head engaging the nurses within his/her department; or it can be an organization-wide approach by a group of like-minded leaders. Regardless of the scope pursued, rest assured that this practice will have a meaningful impact on you as a leader and will catch the attention and imagination of the nurses around you.

# CHAPTER 21

# Support Information for the Conversations

Suggested Questions

Once you start, your personal caring language will identify itself. Consider using prompts that resonate with you.

- Tell me about you.
- Tell me what brings meaning in your work.
- How often do you experience a sense of purpose and meaning?
  - o   What creates those moments?
- When did you last feel like you made a difference?
  - o   What did it involve? How did you feel? What are your thoughts?
- What actions bring meaning to your patients?
- How do real connections happen between you and a patient?
- What do you think about when it comes to authentic caring?

- How do you fit patient connection into your busy shifts?
- What holds you back from feeling authentic—that real connection?
- What is your favorite self-care practice?
  o Tell me about it. How does it impact your caring and your work?

## Caring Language—Its Utility

Language is a method of communication by words and expression used and understood by a community. Human consciousness emerged with the development of language. Language adds dimension to our thoughts and understanding and allows perspective taking. Nursing certainly has its language, but use of a caring language is more recent. Caring language is built from the words of nursing's human caring processes.

Caring words and language come from our caring education, knowledge, and experiences. Caring language is not a foreign language; it's just underutilized in our work environments. Nurses often feel isolated in their authentic caring practices, struggling alone to integrate it into their workloads. Using caring literate words when helping nurses name their caring thoughts, feelings, and behaviors is grounding. Caring is a personal practice and is built from within. Use of caring language expands perspective taking and cultivates consciousness. Using caring language in the conversations, however briefly and episodically, helps validate authentic caring for nurses and nurse leaders and unites us.

## List of Caring Literate Words

- Active listening
- Authenticity—authentic presence
- Authentic caring
- Caring connections
- Connectedness—human connections
- Empathy
- Feelings—not to be judged, denied, or supplanted
- Forgiveness, offering gratitude, surrendering, overcoming fear and pride
- Genuine concern for others
- Humanity—human condition. We are all part of the human condition.
- Inner resources
- Intentionality
- Kindness
- Nonjudgment
- Positive gestures, paying attention
- Reflects on feelings, thoughts, emotions, experiences
- Helps others reflect on their feelings of fear, judgment, loss, trauma
- Respect for self and others
- Self-care practices—cultivate inner resources and mind-body-spirit health
- Self-awareness, self-acceptance, self-compassion
- Pause/silence/reflection
- Vulnerability—recognizing vulnerability in others and in ourselves
- Wellness, well-being

## Caring Literacy—Its Benefits

Literacy is beyond the ability to read and write. It's the ability to understand the basic elements and interconnecting parts of a subject. Literacy basics include definitions, mechanics, and sources. Having literacy in any topic influences behaviors, relationships, and decisions.

Caring literacy is the capacity to obtain, communicate, process, and understand basic information about caring. Caring literacy is an essential component in the fabric of nursing. Sharing and building caring literacy gives nurse leaders words, concepts, and perspectives that can help nurses grow their purpose and meaning in caring. As caring literacy grows, it influences caring behaviors, relationships, and consciousness.

## Caring Literacy Information

**Authentic Caring:** Authentic caring is the essence of nursing. It is the highest level of caring between a nurse and another. This level of caring is where the nurse leads with authenticity and intentionality in caring for a patient, and a deep energy connection occurs that is life-giving and life-receiving for both. Authentic caring moments can impact patients' lives in lasting ways and renew nurses' commitment to their work. Authenticity is a willingness to open oneself up and be present to and accepting of another's feelings, experiences, and vulnerabilities. Authentic caring does not happen in a vacuum; it requires cultivation of nurses' inner resources.

**Authentic Caring Arc:** Reflecting on the interconnecting elements that contribute to the dynamics of authentic caring is informative to nurses. The following description of the arc illustrates the basics: The authentic caring arc originates within the nurse, is sparked by a connection with another, is sustained by the nurses' inner resources and caring consciousness, and has the ability to motivate nurses to remain in nursing by intrinsically rewarding them through their work. The useful aspect in this caring arc illustration is the importance of inner resources and caring consciousness and the role self-care plays in cultivating them.

**Caring Consciousness:** Caring consciousness is our awareness of our thoughts and perceptions around caring. Consciousness is how we are aware of thoughts. Language is a critical element in consciousness cultivation (Hayes 2016).[53]

**Caring Relationships:** Reflecting on the distinctions of the five levels of caring relationships provides a context and understanding of nurses' caring experiences. Understanding the levels expands self-awareness and caring consciousness. The Five Basic Levels of Caring Relationships are: 1) Life-destroying (biocidic)—the nurse causes distress for a patient by depersonalizing and increasing vulnerability. 2) Life-restraining (biostatic)—the nurse is insensitive or indifferent to the other, creating uneasiness. 3) Life-neutral (biopassive)—where nursing care is no more than a job, and there is little regard for the patient's circumstance. 4) Life-sustaining (bioactive)—a nurse who is kind, concerned, reassuring, and responsive to patients' needs. This level has become the baseline standard for nursing care in organizations. 5) Life-giving (biogenic)—this is the level of an authentic caring connection. This connection relieves the patient's vulnerability and is life-giving and life-receiving for both the nurse and patient (Halldorsdottir 1991).[34] This is considered a transpersonal caring relationship (Watson 2012).[35]

**Caring Science:** There are varied definitions of caring science. One definition from Florida Atlantic University Christine E. Lynn College of Nursing describes caring science as a body of knowledge, based on theory and research, that focuses on the relationship of caring to health, healing, and well-being of the whole person within the context of family, community, and environment. Another definition of caring science describes it as the science of caring; grounded in humanity and the ethics of belonging; expanding beyond medical science and acknowledging the relational, life forces that underlie all of humanity (Turkel, Watson, and Giovannoni 2018).[54]

**Humanity:** Humanity is humankind—all human beings collectively. Humanity is the quality of being humane. The human condition is all things that can happen in life and leave humans in vulnerable situations. Nursing responds to the human condition and those humans caught in vulnerable situations. Nurses' sense of humanity embodies not only sensitivity to the human condition but also acceptance and nonjudgment of the people experiencing the condition.

**Individualism:** Maintaining a consistent sense of humanity is difficult in Western societies that are strongly based on individualism (Johnson 2018).[55] Our culture's groupthink is that each of us is responsible for ourselves. We expect every person to be doing his/her best, even those who are struggling and suffering, such as our patients. The side effect of individualism is that other peoples' "best" may not meet our expectations, and before we know it, we are judging individuals for the situation they are in—the human condition they are experiencing. This is rampant in the health care system, where many illnesses, diseases, traumas are considered lifestyle choices—substance abuse, mental illness, incarceration, obesity, chronic diseases, etc. This groupthink is hard to counter for the individual nurse. Leadership that demonstrates consistent nonjudgmental messages and behaviors is the best antidote. Seeing patients—and all people—in the context of the human condition diminishes the power of individualism.

**Inner Resources:** Inner resources are those thoughts and emotions that feed our sense of self, self-awareness, self-acceptance, self-compassion, and self-love. "We have to offer caring, love, forgiveness, (gratitude), compassion and mercy to ourselves in order to offer authentic caring and love to others" (Watson 2008, 41).[56] For nurses, job stress and inner stress trigger self-protection, limit access to our authenticity, and stifle our ability to engage and connect with patients in meaningful ways. Finding fulfillment in nursing requires self-care with its self-healing capacities to open the door of authenticity and meaningful connection with others in our work.

**Intrinsic Motivators:** An intrinsic motivator is an internal reward generated by the performance of something. It has three essential elements: autonomy—the desire to direct our own lives; mastery—the urge to make progress and get better at something that matters; and purpose—the yearning to do what we do in the service of something larger than ourselves (Pink 2009, 219).[29]

**Naming Feelings, Behaviors, Experiences:** Helping others name their feelings, behaviors, and experiences that arise in their caring process provides clarification and is a critical component in discovery. The process of translating an event with a simple word or label helps raise awareness and anchors the understanding. I first learned the importance of helping others name events from that parenting book I used when my girls were young. Since then that parenting book became a leadership book for me (Faber and Mazlish 2012).[8] The benefits of naming feelings, behaviors, and experiences have been reinforced in coaching literature (Miller and Rollnick 2013),[57] in mindfulness literature (Hanson 2016),[58] and in compassionate communications literature (Rosenberg 2015).[59] In fact, Rosenberg, a psychologist and creator of nonviolent communication, describes needs and feelings as fundamentally linked. Meeting people's needs is certainly important, but it's in the process of knowing that one's feelings are being heard is where the healing occurs. I saw this as a nurse leader; once nurses' feelings were authentically heard with no judgment or correction, the possibilities of self-discovery opened up.

**Vulnerability:** "Vulnerability is not a weakness, and the uncertainty, risk, and emotional exposure we face every day are not optional. Our choice is a question of engagement. Our willingness to own and engage with our vulnerability determines the depth of our courage and the clarity of our purpose; the level to which we protect ourselves from being vulnerable is a measure of our fear and disconnection" (Brown 2012, 2).[12] As nurses, we see patients experiencing life vulnerabilities every day in our work, and it can trigger our own fears of being vulnerable.

Vulnerability experiences—in our own lives—are the main thing that holds us back from letting go of control and self-protection. Depending on our level of self-protection in any moment, determines our level of authenticity and full engagement with others. For nurses, job stress and inner stress trigger self-protection and impact our ability to access our authenticity and our ability to engage and connect with patients in meaningful ways.

**Wellness Consciousness:** Wellness consciousness is our awareness of our state of wellness and all that contributes to it. Wellness consciousness encompasses the recognition that health isn't just absence of disease and illness; it's mind-body-spirit health. Wellness is a state of being, a journey, a way of living toward achieving one's full potential. Wellness is a dynamic process that takes into account all the factors that contribute to well-being. The ten dimensions of wellness are physical, nutritional, medical and dental, social, environmental, spiritual, behavioral and intellectual, psychological, occupational, and financial. Wellness practices are self-care practices. Well-being is the state in which we enjoy positive emotions and relationships, feel satisfied with life, and live a fulfilling, meaningful life (Institute of Wellness Education 2016).[60]

# CONCLUSION: SAVING NURSES

Authentic caring certainly exists today but not at the frequency or systemic level it could if it was a conscious and visible part of our work environments. The essence of nursing is authentic caring. Authentic caring has always been the central anchor of nursing's contribution to health care and society. And now society's wellness renaissance is shifting expectations of health care closer into alignment with nursing caring science. In addition, patient experience metrics are reflecting patients' recognition of the health and healing powers of nurses' authentic caring connections. "Caring consciousness skills are as critical as clinical skills to patients' well-being, nurses' caring connections, healthcare's organizational cultures, and society's wellness" (McClendon 2017, 41).[61]

This shift in alignment and recognition of nursing comes at a time when nurses' authentic caring capacity is waning. Nurse attrition evidence indicates that nearly half of the population of new nurses may be looking for ways to leave nursing. The reality is that the pace and complexity in nurses' jobs leave too many nurses feeling alone and disconnected from their original purpose in being a nurse. How nurse leaders within the health care industry locally and at large address this nurse condition and nursing attrition is the challenge before us. It is not just about job satisfaction; it is about nurses thriving in nursing. Creative cultivation of collateral pathways is needed to help more nurses stay in nursing. While the majority of retention efforts focus on mitigating job and environmental stressors that drive nurses out of nursing, equal time and effort must be given to what keeps nurses in nursing. There is a lot of territory to cover. Nurses learning to thrive in nursing can offset attrition. The mission is to expand caring consciousness cultivation at the grassroots level for more nurses beyond the current reach.

Understanding these contextual forces brings nurse leaders to a new territory, one of seeing their roles anew. This is a big hurdle. Nurse leaders are already stretched beyond capacity. Nurses need help, and so do nurse leaders. Through this book, nurse leaders can hopefully see the complexity of their roles more clearly and feel better about themselves, knowing that they are not alone. By telling my story, I hope other nurse leaders will see their stories and new caring cultivation pathways to be created in their world.

How nurse leaders lead caring impacts how caring is recognized, understood, and valued by all within the health care industry. Nurse leaders giving voice to authentic caring and engaging with nurses in caring discovery and cultivation is one step forward in helping nurses learn to thrive in nursing. This will save nurses from leaving nursing. This can be nurse leaders' twenty-first-century legacy.

# Notes

1   Jean Watson, *Postmodern Nursing and Beyond* (Edinburgh: Churchill Livingstone,1999),46.

2   Andrea Kabcenell, Jessica Perlo, and Bonnie R. Sakallaris, "Joy in Work: Creating Fulfilled, Productive Health Care Teams," *AONE, Voice of Nursing Leadership*, (November 2016): 4–6

3   Carol Isaac MacKusick and Ptiene Minick, "Why Are Nurses Leaving? Findings from an Initial Qualitative Study on Nursing Attrition," *MEDSURG Nursing* 19, no. 6 (November/December 2010): 335–40.

4   Nora E. Warshawsky and Donna S. Havens, "Nurse Manager Job Satisfaction and Intent to Leave," *Nursing Economics* 32, no. 1 (2010): 32–9.

5   Susan Levi, Lisa Montgomery, and Eileen Hurd, "The Colorado Differentiated Practice Model," *Nursing Management* 25, no. 10 (October 1994): 54.

6   Jim Collins, *Good To Great* (New York: Harper Business, 2001). Collins's point that being good is the enemy of achieving greatness is a human problem. It requires facing brutal facts and the discipline of people, thoughts, and actions to rise beyond the level of being good.

7   Magnet Recognition Program
    The Magnet Recognition Program is a recognition program operated by the American Nurses Credentialing Center that allows nurses to recognize nursing excellence in other nurses. It is considered the highest recognition for nursing excellence.

https://www.nursingworld.org/organizational-programs/magnet/

8   Adele Faber and Elaine Mazlish, *How to Talk So Kids Will Listen and Listen So Kids Will Talk* (New York: Avon Books, 2012 edition), 1–46.

9   Bill Moyers, "Healing and the Mind," *National Public Radio documentary series*, 1993.

10  Emmett Murphy, "Leadership IQ in Hospitals," Keynote presentation, September 2000, *VHA Conference Leadership*, Dallas Texas.

11  Fred Lee. "If Disney Ran Your Hospital." Keynote presentation, October 2006, Community Hospital Annual Leadership Conference, Colorado.

12  Brene Brown, *Daring Greatly* (New York: Penguin Books, 2012).
    Falling in the arena refers to those facedown moments were a person fails and everyone is watching.

13  Value-Based Purchasing (VBP) Program
    The Hospital Value-Based Purchasing (VBP) Program is a Centers for Medicare and Medicaid Services (CMS) initiative that affects the payment structure for inpatient stays in hospitals across the country. Payments are based on quality care measurements, one of which is patient satisfaction, which strongly correlates with nursing care quality indicators. This adds more pressures on nursing leaders' performance.

14  DAISY Foundation Award
    An acronym for Diseases Attacking the Immune System, The DAISY Foundation was formed in November, 1999, by the family of J. Patrick Barnes, who died at age thirty-three of complications of idiopathic thrombocytopenic purpura (ITP). The nursing care Patrick received when hospitalized profoundly touched his family.
    https://www.daisyfoundation.org/daisy-award

15  Press Ganey Associates
    Press Ganey is one of the CMS (Centers for Medicare & Medicaid Services) designated organizations that collect and

report patient satisfaction data for hospitals. Press Ganey Associates is also a health care consulting organization focusing on safety, quality, and patient experience.

16  Diana M. Crowell. "Leadership In Complex Nursing and Health Care Systems," in *Nursing, Caring, and Complexity Science For Human-Environment Well-Being,* eds. Alice Ware Davidson, Marilyn A. Ray, and Marian C. Turkel (New York: Springer Publishing Company; 2011), 199–211.

17  Alice Ware Davidson, Marilyn A. Ray, and Marian C. Turkel, eds., *Nursing, Caring, and Complexity Science For Human-Environment Well-Being* (New York: Springer Publishing Company, 2011).

18  Patricia Liehr and Mary Jane Smith. "Modeling the Complexity of Story Theory for Nursing Practice," in *Nursing, Caring, and Complexity Science For Human-Environment Well-Being,* eds. Alice Ware Davidson, Marilyn A. Ray, Marian C. Turkel (New York: Springer Publishing Company; 2011), 241–48.

Story theory is a framework to develop a patient's story. It is a narrative of reflections and meaning the patient gives to their health challenge.

19  Robert Wood Johnson Foundation (RWJF)

The RWJF is a large philanthropic organization solely dedicated to health and the health care system. They are a major funder of health care research, education, improvements, and advocacy.

20  The Institute of Medicine (IOM) is affiliated with the National Academies of Science and serves as a nonprofit organization devoted to leadership on health care. In 2016 the IOM was renamed the Health and Medicine Division (HMD) of the National Academies.

21  "The Future of Nursing: Leading Change, Advancing Health," Institute of Medicine report in 2010, accessed September 9, 2018,
https://www.ncbi.nlm.nih.gov/pubmed/24983041

22  Joyce E. Johnson, Teresa Veneziano, Tracey Malast, Kari Mastro, Annloise Moran, Lori Mulligan, Amy L. Smith,

"Nursing's Future: What's the message?" *Nursing Management* 43, no.7 (July 2012); 37-41.

23　"The State of Nursing 2016—White Paper," by Nursing.org, Bureau of Labor Statistics (BLS), July 2016, accessed May 15, 2018,
www.nursing.org/wp-content/uploads/ ... /Nursing.org_. State-of-Nursing_2016.pdf

24　Tim Porter-O'Grady, Marilyn A. Hawkins and Marsha L. Parker, *Whole-Systems Shared Governance: Architecture for Integration* (Maryland: An Aspen Publication, 1997).
American Nurses Credentialing Center: ANCC Magnet Recognition Program,
https://www.nursingworld.org/organizational-programs/ magnet/.
American Nurses Credentialing Center: ANCC Pathway to Excellence Program,
https://www.nursingworld.org/organizational-programs/ pathway/.
Robert Wood Johnson Foundation: Transforming Care at the Bedside Program,
https://www.rwjf.org/en/library/research/2011/07/ transforming-care-at-the-bedside.html.

25　The Advisory Board is a private organization that acts as a "think tank" focusing on health care and the performance health care organizations. They generate research and technology and consult with health care organizations.

26　Jenna Koppel, Katherine Virkstis, Sarah Strumwasser, Marie Katz, Carol Boston-Fleischhauer, "Regulating the Flow of Change to Reduce Frontline Nurse Stress and Burnout," *Journal of Nursing Administration* 45, no. 11, (2015): 534–36.

27　"Ask, Affirm, Assess, Act—The 4A's to Rise Above Moral Distress," American Association Critical-Care Nurses (AACN), 2009, accessed October 3, 2018, https://www.emergingrnleader.com/wp-content/ uploads/2012/06/4As_to_Rise_Above_Moral_Distress.pdf

28  Arnold Baker and Wilmar B. Schaufeli, "The Utrecht Work Engagement Scale (UWES)," accessed October 3, 2018, https://www.researchgate.net/publication/312805574_The_Utrecht_Work_Engagement_Scale_UWES_Test_manual.

29  Daniel Pink, *Drive: The Surprising Truth About What Motivates Us* (New York: Riverhead Books, 2009).

30  The Institute of Healthcare Improvement (IHI) is an independent not-for-profit organization that leads innovative healthcare improvement worldwide through partnerships. www.ihi.org/

31  Lynn Greenleaf Brown, Tanya L. Johnson, Libba Reed McMillan, and Amy Brandon, "Two Heads Are Better Than One—Partnering to Improve a Critical Care Work Environment," *Nursing Management* 49, no.7 (July 2018): 23–29

32  Jessica Perlo, Barbara Balik, Stephen Swensen, Andrea Kabcenell, Julie Landsman, and Derek Feeley. "IHI Framework for Improving Joy in Work," White Paper by Institute for Healthcare Improvement, 2017, Cambridge, Massachusetts, http://www.ihi.org/Topics/Joy-In-Work/Pages/default.aspx

33  Lee Galuska, Judith Hahn, E. Carol Polifroni, and Gregory Crow, A Narrative Analysis of Nurses' Experiences With Meaning and Joy in Nursing Practice. *Nursing Administration Quarterly*2, no. 2 (2018): 154–63.

34  Sigridur Halldorsdottir, "Five Basic Modes of Being With Another," in *Caring: The Compassionate Healer*, eds. Delores A. Gaut and Madeleine M. Leininger (New York: National League for Nursing Press,1991), 37–49.

35  Jean Watson, *Human Caring Science* Second edition. (Sudbury, MA: Jones & Bartlett Learning, 2012).

36  Darlene Amendolair, "Caring Behaviors and Job Satisfaction," *Journal of Nursing Administration* 42, no.1 (2012): 34–39

37  Michael J. Dotson, Dinesh S. Dave, Joseph A. Cazier, and Trent J. Spaulding, "An Empirical Analysis of Nurse Retention," *Journal of Nursing Administration* 44, no. 2 (2014): 111–16.

38  Kelly Kester and Holly Wei, "Building Nurse Resilience," *Nursing Management* 49, no.6 (June 2018): 42–45.

39  Donna L Magtibay, Sherry S. Chesak, Kevin Coughlin, and Amit Sood, "Decreasing Stress and Burnout in Nurses," *Journal of Nursing Administration* 47, no. 7/8, (2017): 391–95.

40  Jean Watson, "Caring Science and Caritas Processes," presentation in online class: Caring Science, Mindful Practice, January 2016, *Canvas Network*.

41  Margie Eckroth-Bucher, "Self-Awareness: A Review and Analysis of a Basic Nursing Concept," *Advances in Nursing Science* 33, no. 4 (2010): 297–309.

42  Sharon J. Tucker, Audrey J. Weymiller, Suzanne M. Cutshall, Lori M. Rhudy, and Christine M. Lohse, "Stress Ratings and Health Promotion Practices Among RNs: A Case For Action," *Journal of Nursing Administration* 42, no. 5 (2012): 282–92.

43  Kathleen Neville and Donna A. Cole, "The Relationships Among Health Promotion Behaviors, Compassion Fatigue, Burnout, and Compassion Satisfaction in Nurses Practicing in a Community Medical Center," *Journal of Nursing Administration* 43, no. 6 (2013): 348–54.

44  Heather L. Williams, Teresa Costley, Lanell M. Bellury, and Jasmine Moobed, "Do Health Promotion Behaviors Affect Levels of Job Satisfaction and Job Stress for Nurses in an Acute Care Hospital?" *Journal of Nursing Administration* 48, no. 6 (June 2018): 342–48.

45  Maggie McCright, Christine Pabico, and Nikki Roux, "Addressing Manager Retention with the Pathway to Excellence Framework," *Nursing Management* 49, no.8 (August 2018): 6–8.

46  Susan MacLeod Dyess, Angela S. Prestia, and Marlaine C. Smith, "*Support for Caring and Resiliency Among Successful Nurse Leaders*," *Nursing Administration Quarterly* 39, no. 2 (2015): 104–16.

47  Watson Caring Science Institute (WCSI), https://www.watsoncaringscience.org/
Watson Caring Science Institute offers education and programs that inform and inspire the use of Dr. Jean Watson's theory

of human caring/caring science. These programs guide transformative models of caring and healing practices for hospitals, nurses, and patients in diverse settings worldwide. There is a range of online programs available.

48  American Holistic Nurses Association (AHNA) https://www. ahna.org/

49  Caritas Coach Education Program (CCEP)–offered through WCSI.
    ,https://www.watsoncaringscience.org/.
    This is a unique, extensive, six-month, semistructured program designed specifically for caring consciousness cultivation. It is an experiential, aesthetic, personal, ethical, and intellectual journey into caring science praxis.
    I am forever grateful for the wisdom of the Caritas coach leaders and Caritas coaches.

50  Virginia M. Mason, Gail Leslie, Kathleen Clark, Pat Lyons, Erica Walke, Christina Butler, and Martha Griffin, "Compassion Fatigue, Moral Distress, and Work Engagement in Surgical Intensive Care Unit Trauma Nurses," *Dimensions of Critical Care Nursing* 33, no. 4 (July/Aug 2014): 215–25.

51  Chris Witherspoon, "Oprah Discusses How Maya Angelou Helped To Define Her Legacy," theGrio, May 28, 2014, https://thegrio.com/2014/05/28/maya-angelou-dead-oprah-legacy/

52  James R. Doty, "Alphabet of the Heart: 10 Steps Along the Journey Towards Compassion and Mindfulness," Keynote presentation*: 23ʳᵈ International Caritas Consortium Conference*, October 26.2017, Watson Caring Science Center & Stanford Health Care.

53  Steve C. Hayes, Perspective-Taking As Healing, in *the Self-Acceptance Project*, (ed.) Tami Simon (Boulder: Sounds True, 2016), 27–36.

54  Marian C. Turkel, Jean Watson, and Joseph Giovannoni, "Caring Science or Science of Caring," *Nursing Science Quarterly* 3, no. 1 (2018): 66–71.

55 Allan G. Johnson, *Privilege, Power, and Difference* Third Edition (New York: McGraw Hill, 2018).

56 Jean Watson, *The Philosophy and Science of Caring* (Boulder: University Press of Colorado, 2008).

57 William R. Miller and Stephen Rollnick, *Motivational Interviewing: Helping People Change* Third Edition (New York: The Guilford Press, 2013).

58 Rick Hanson, Taking in the Good, in *the Self-Acceptance Project*, (ed.) Tami Simon (Boulder: Sounds True, 2016), 125–32.

59 Marshall B. Rosenberg, *Nonviolent Communication* (Encinitas: Puddle Dancer Press, 2015).

60 Institute of Wellness Education, "Wellness Coaching Level 1 Certification Program," 2016, Department of Labor's Registered Apprenticeship in Wellness Coaching. https://www.instituteforwellness.com/about/

61 Pat McClendon, "Authentic Caring: Rediscover the Essence of Nursing," *Nursing Management* 48, no.10 (October 2017): 39.

# Resources

Boykin, Anne and Savina O. Schoenhofer, 2013. *Nursing As Caring: A Model for Transforming Practice.* EBook: National League of Nursing Press.

Dossey, Barbara Montgomery, Susan Luck, and Bonney Gulino Schaub, 2015. *Nurse Coaching: Integrative Approaches for Health and Wellbeing.* North Miami: International Nurse Coach Association.

Lee, Susan M., Patrick A. Palmieri, and Jean Watson, eds. 2017. *Global Advances in Human Caring Literacy.* New York: Springer Publishing Company.

Horton-Deutsch, Sara, and Jan Anderson, eds. 2018. *Caritas Coaching: A Journey Towards Transpersonal Cairn for Informed Moral Action in Health care.* Indianapolis, IN: Sigma Theta Tau International.

Madril, Eddie, Sara Moncada, and Kathy Douglas. 2015. *The Dance of Caring: A Caregiver's Guide to Harmony* Wavena, Inc.: www.TheDanceofCaring.com

Porter-O'Grady, Tim and Kathy Malloch. 2011. *Quantum Leadership* Third ed. Sudbury, MA: Jones & Bartlett Learning.

Sherwood, Gwen D. and Sara Horton-Deutsch. 2012. *Reflective Practice: Transforming Education and Improving Outcomes.* Indianapolis, IN: Sigma Theta Tau International.

Sitzman, Kathleen and Jean Watson. 2014. Caring Science, Mindful Practice. New York: Springer Publishing Company.

CPSIA information can be obtained
at www.ICGtesting.com
Printed in the USA
FSHW012104110419
57176FS